Make Weight Loss Last

Deborah Kesten is the author of:

The Healing Secrets of Food

Feeding the Body, Nourishing the Soul

Make Weight Loss Last

10 Solutions That Nourish Body, Mind, and Soul

Deborah Kesten, M.P.H.
Larry Scherwitz, PH.D.

White River Press
Amherst, Massachusetts

Make Weight Loss Last: 10 Solutions That Nourish Body, Mind, and Soul
Copyright © 2012 by Deborah Kesten and Larry Scherwitz

First published 2007 as *The Englightened Diet: 7 Weight-Loss Solutions That Nourish Body, Mind, and Soul,* Celestial Arts/Ten Speed Press/Random House

Expanded, updated edition published 2012 by White River Press

White River Press
PO Box 3561
Amherst, MA 01004
www.whiteriverpress.com

Cover design by Rebecca Niemark, twenty-six letters

Library of Congress Cataloging-in-Publication Data

Kesten, Deborah, 1948–
Make weight loss last: 10 solutions that nourish body, mind and soul / Deborah Kesten, Larry Scherwitz.
           p.   cm.
Rev. ed. of: Enlightened diet / Deborah Kesten and Larry Scherwitz. c2007.
ISBN 978-1-935052-61-6 (pbk. : alk. paper) — ISBN 978-1-887043-05-2 (ebook)
          1. Weight loss. 2. Reducing diets. 3. Nutrition. I. Scherwitz, Larry.
          II. Kesten, Deborah, 1948– Enlightened diet. III. Title.
          RM222.2.K48 2012
          613.2'5—dc23
          2012014992

Preface to the New Edition

I t's regrettable that effective ways to lose weight and keep it off have remained a mystery for so long. Most of us know more about what *doesn't* work for the long term: dieting and magical quick–fix solutions that promise overnight success. We're paying a big price for our ignorance, and for the illusion that losing weight is easy. Not only do millions of us struggle with our growing girth, but we also experience immense frustration when we regain the weight it took so long to lose.

Have you considered that there might be more than just one or two ways—eat less, exercise more—to lose weight and keep it off? Most of us haven't. Did you know that teamwork—using a "family" of strategies (often unfamiliar ones)—can increase your chances of success? Most of us don't. This updated and expanded edition of *Make Weight Loss Last* reveals ten reasons we're overweight and offers ten solutions for both losing weight and keeping it off.

In the original version of this book, published in 2007 as *The Enlightened Diet,*[1] we talked a lot about seven of those ten reasons— the "eating styles" our original research had linked with overeating, overweight, and obesity. We call these Food Fretting, Task Snacking, Emotional Eating, Fast Foodism, Solo Dining, Unappetizing Atmosphere, and Sensory Disregard.[2] The seven eating styles emerged when we took a step back and compared what and how people had eaten for thousands of years[3,4] to today's "new normal" of fast food, emotional eating, dieting, dining alone, and eating on the run—often in unpleasant atmospheres, and without taking the time to truly taste our food. The bottom line: *not only are the seven overeating styles the new normal way of eating, they're all linked to overeating, overweight, and obesity.*

Since identifying these overeating styles, we've come to realize this simple fact about why so many of us struggle with weight: the more we veer away from the life−giving properties of food and the multidimensional ways in which it nourished us for millennia, the more we're likely to be overweight or obese, and the less we're likely to be able to lose weight and keep it off.

We're deeply concerned about how today's cultural landscape has reshaped us. After all, today's typical American fare and *how* we eat (often quickly, distracted, alone) weren't our "eating styles" as we evolved as human beings. In *Make Weight Loss Last*, we'll show you how the seven eating styles affect weight. And we'll explain how three other "new normals"—hidden chemicals in food, inadequate sleep, and not enough exercise—can cause you to pack on pounds and make it hard to lose them.

At its core, *Make Weight Loss Last* is sounding the siren to halt and reverse the relatively recent cultural shift, the new normal of time−saving, chemical−laden cuisine and inadequate sleep and exercise—trends that are unequivocally contributing to our growing girth. We offer insights and solutions that, until now, have eluded many of us. Reaping the rewards calls for reclaiming our food—and healthy−weight—heritage. In this way, *Make Weight Loss Last* may help you transform your relationship to food, eating, and weight, and in the process find true nourishment.

Table of Contents

"The key to [weight loss] success is maintenance and changing what and how you eat."

—Gayle King, Anchor, *CBS This Morning*[1]

Introduction

Make Weight Loss Last: The 10 Solutions

W hy are some people far more successful than others at losing weight and keeping it off ? The persistent story about those who succeed at weight loss focuses on eating less and moving more. But the true ingredients of weight loss success are more complex, and if you want to understand how to lose weight and keep it off, look to ancient food wisdom and merge that with insights from modern nutritional science. You'll discover such weight–control "secrets" as fresh food, dining with others, even tasting and appreciating food. During our careers as health researchers, the nutrition journey we've taken around the world has shown the elements that make weight loss last to be far more multifaceted—and remarkable—than we've been led to believe.

In 1980 in America, 43 percent of Americans were overweight and obese. In the space of less than thirty years, from 1980 to 2009, the numbers of overweight and obese Americans jumped dramati–cally. If you were to look at the increase on a graph, the line would rise sharply, so much so that today 68 percent of adults are overweight or obese,[2] as are one–third of children and adolescents.[3, 4] And 32 percent of *infants* are obese or at risk for obesity.[5]

What has caused America's rates of obesity to skyrocket? The easy explanation is that many Americans are consuming more calories than their bodies need. But is the answer really so simple?

According to the U.S. Centers for Disease Control and Prevention (CDC), most of the excess calories we're consuming come from a

Are You Overweight or Obese?

Overweight and obesity are labels that describe an abnormal or excessive amount of fat accumulation. While the number on the scale was used for decades to determine if you're overweight or obese, the Body mass index (BMI) is the new gold standard for measuring weight and height to calculate a person's amount of body fat. To classify overweight or obesity in adults, the BMI measures weight in kilograms divided by the square of a person's height in meters (kg/m^2).

Here are BMI guidelines that correlate with a person's amount of body fat:

- underweight: 18.5
- healthy weight: 18.5 to 24.9
- overweight: 25.0 to 29.9
- obesity: 30 or higher

Because the degree of body fat differs from person to person, BMI is considered a rough guide to determine overweight or obesity. It does not directly measure body fat. Other methods of estimating body fat and body fat distribution include measure—ments of skinfold thickness, waist circumference, waist—to—hip circumference ratios, and technology such as ultrasound, computed tomography (CT scan), and magnetic resonance imaging (MRI).

fast—food diet high in fats, carbohydrates, and calories; add a sed—entary lifestyle, and you have a formula for weight gain. In other words, conventional wisdom says that fast food and lack of exercise are the two key causes of today's raging obesity epidemic. Given that Americans are eating more while physical education is no longer required in schools and exercise has been squeezed out by work, family responsibilities, and television and video games, the explana—

tion that there's an imbalance between calories consumed and calo—ries burned makes sense.[6]

But Ashley N. Gearhardt and team members affiliated with Yale University's Rudd Center for Obesity Food Policy and Research offer another reason: food addiction. For decades, many people with food issues suspected their struggle had something to do with a force that was out of their control—in the same way that substances such as cocaine, chemicals in cigarettes, or compulsive behaviors such as gambling and shopping are addictive.

Recent research published in the *Archives of General Psychiatry* vindicates those whose beliefs were previously dismissed. It's offi—cial: food addiction is real. When study participants filled out the Yale Food Addiction Scale (YFAS), those with the higher food addiction scores showed greater activation in areas of the brain linked with sub—stance dependence. In other words, addictive—like eating behavior (in response to food cues) and substance dependence activate the same reward circuitry in the brain. "To our knowledge, this is the first study to link indicators of addictive eating behavior with a specific pattern of neural activation," Gearhardt says. "This may partially explain the difficulty people experience in achieving sustainable weight loss."[7] Gearhardt's food—addiction findings suggest that healthful foods and exercise bring benefits, but they're not necessarily effective solutions for sustained weight loss. People who struggle with food addiction may profit more from a comprehensive treatment program, perhaps in a residential setting.

A third major theory about the cause of obesity is based on endo—crinology, the branch of medicine that deals with disorders of the endocrine glands and hormones. According to this medical specialty, obesity doesn't always stem from behavioral issues such as overeating, underexercising, or food addictions. Endocrine researchers are leading exciting research about physiological factors (such as genetic prob—lems) and internal mechanisms (hormonal imbalances, for instance) that control how food is metabolized, how appetite is generated, and how a sense of satiety is experienced. They are asking such ques—tions as, "Does genetics determine how we use and burn energy? Do particular hormones affect how calories are processed? Might other systems in the body affect appetite?" By taking such questions into account when working with obese patients, some physicians are addressing considerations that go beyond diet and exercise.

All three of these explanations are rational, accurate, and relevant. Each attributes a different dynamic to today's obesity problem; at the same time, all three share the viewpoint that something has changed in our relatively recent past that has tipped overeating and obesity into a relentless—and worsening—epidemic. In other words, changes in our external and internal environments over the last few decades— what we consume, how much we eat or exercise, even our genes and hormones—may all be working together to make us fat.

Our own research has identified yet more changes in our relationship with food over the last few decades. These changes are so profound that they alter not only weight and physical health but also psychological, spiritual, and social well-being. We call these "new normal" ways of eating the "seven overeating styles." And they all appear to powerfully influence your weight in different ways.

A New View

We are researchers who specialize in preventing and reversing obesity and heart disease through diet and other lifestyle building blocks, such as stress management, strong social support, physical activity, and more. We've conducted large clinical trials in both the United States and Europe to discover the "best" way to eat and live in order to promote a health-filled life. [8,9] Given our passion for using evidence-based, sound science to help others enhance health and achieve wellness, we've felt frustration as America's battle with obesity has continued to escalate.

We feel particularly sad about the excessive extra weight so many of us struggle with, because being overweight or obese significantly increases the risk not only of developing a chronic condition—from heart disease and diabetes to high blood pressure and more—but also of dying from it. As we write, more than two-thirds of Americans are either overweight or obese, and for the first time in two centuries, the life expectancy of the younger generation is projected to be shorter than that of their parents—because of the ever−growing number of overweight children, teens, *and infants.*[10]

Would it be possible to create an evidence−based, *sustainable* program that could help people achieve normal weight as part of a pleasurable and normal way of life—not as a restricted regimen that starts, stops, and often ends in failure? As we considered this, we realized that prior to the obesity epidemic that has emerged in the last few decades, most Americans—indeed, most people worldwide—were of normal weight. What, we wondered, had worked for so many of us for so many centuries?

Back to the Future
Sometimes you have to go backward before you can move forward. The research we'd done previously with heart patients provided clues to what might work, because it had opened our eyes to the astounding healing potential of one of the oldest health−and−healing programs on the planet: the yogic lifestyle. We were very familiar with the healing power of yoga, because co−author Larry Scherwitz was the director of research for more than eighteen years with pioneering physician Dr. Dean Ornish, whose repeated studies showed that heart disease could be reversed through yoga−based lifestyle changes (diet, exercise, stress management, social support)—without drugs or surgery.[11] Co−author Deborah Kesten was the nutritionist on Dr. Ornish's first clinical trial for reversing heart disease,[8] as well as director of nutrition on similar research at cardiovascular clinics in Europe.[12]

Our in−depth understanding of the ancient yogic lifestyle inspired us to go beyond today's typical nutritional prescription of what and how much to eat in order to lose weight. As we mulled over the concept, it became clear to us that we could create a comprehensive blueprint for eating to achieve optimal weight by merging modern nutritional science with ancient food wisdom—from world religions, cultural traditions, and healing systems that had provided wise, effective food−and−eating guidelines for millennia. And because traditional dieting doesn't bring lasting weight loss for most of us, our nutrition journey around the world would include what *does* work— as a way of life and eating, *not* as a typical restrictive food regimen.

What we found was astonishing. We discovered a cornucopia of ancient food wisdom that had provided advice about optimal nutrition and eating for centuries before science became the uncontested expert in the twentieth century. It took us more than five years to uncover the best secrets to optimal eating. During our quest, we researched nutrition and food wisdom from Western nutritional science as well as from cultures where people are naturally thinner and healthier, such as the Mediterranean region and France. But we didn't stop there. We investigated timeless food wisdom from Eastern healing systems—traditional Chinese medicine (TCM), India's Ayurvedic principles, and Tibetan medicine.

Excited about our findings, we continued our exploration by analyzing dietary guidelines from world religions (Judaism, Christianity, Islam, Hinduism, Buddhism) and cultural traditions (the yoga diet, Native American food beliefs, African–American soul food, the Japanese Way of Tea, Chinese food folklore). To add yet more substance and understanding, we interviewed more than fifty scientists, and religion and spiritual experts.[13]

Whole Person Nutrition

When we stepped back to reflect on such rich and abundant guidelines from wisdom and cultural traditions and healing systems, six time–tested "secrets" emerged—perennial principles that have served humankind for millennia. Because these themes recurred so often, they can be considered universal guidelines: fresh food, positive feelings, mindfulness, gratitude, love, and socializing.

To make meaning of these themes, we turned them into cohesive guidelines, and when we took a closer look we realized that they encompass the four basic facets of food. They provide guidelines for *biological* (what to eat for physical health), *psychological* (how food affects feelings), *spiritual* (the life–giving meaning in meals), and *social* (dining with others) nourishment. Here's how the six guidelines look from that perspective:

BIOLOGICAL NUTRITION

1. Eat fresh whole foods in their natural state as often as possible.

PSYCHOLOGICAL NUTRITION
2. Be aware of feelings before, during, and after eating.

SPIRITUAL NUTRITION
3. Bring moment–to–moment nonjudgmental awareness to every aspect of the meal.
4. Appreciate food and its origins—from the heart.
5. Create union with the Divine by "flavoring" food with love.

SOCIAL NUTRITION
6. Unite with others through food.

The four facets of food tell us what religions and cultural traditions seemed to know instinctively and intuitively and what modern researchers are beginning to conjecture: that food empowers us to heal multidimensionally. We coined the term "whole person nutrition" to describe the "four facet" way of eating, because the facets empower us to make connections, each time we eat, between food and body, food and mind, food and soul, and food and social well–being.[14,15]

We were excited about our findings, because the guidelines are consistent with what health professionals worldwide recommend (as do caring cooks and all of us who savor good food). But the question remained: would the eating guidelines and food facets weigh in with weight loss—or, conversely, with overeating? In other words, do they have anything to do with how much we weigh?

Our "New Normal": Seven Overeating Styles
To find out if there's a link between perennial food wisdom and weight, we partnered with *Spirituality & Health* magazine. In its cover story on our six guidelines, readers were invited to take our six–week, eighteen lesson e–course (called "The Enlightened Diet") on the magazine's website. Participants first completed an eighty–item whole person nutrition survey and entered their height and weight. Lessons were replete with opportunities to discover, internalize, and practice the whole person nutrition program via workshop–like exercises, "nutritips," discussion groups, and a question–and–answer section.

After the six weeks, participants filled out the survey again. In this way, we were able to see if any changes had occurred in their eating patterns and weight. We were encouraged and inspired by two findings:

- At the start of the study, the 69 percent of the 5,256 participants who were overweight or obese followed the six perennial principles the least. Those within a normal weight range were much closer to following the six principles but still had room for improvement. This told us that the less people adhere to these principles, the more likely they are to be overweight.
- Throughout the e−course, those who increasingly ate according to the six perennial themes were the ones who lost the most weight.[16,17]

While the implications were enormous in relation to the question of how to lose weight, with another turn of our statistical kaleidoscope we realized that the thoughts, feelings, and behaviors elicited by our questionnaire could be clustered into styles of eating. And with this insight, we identified seven specific patterns of eating and problem behaviors that predict overeating and weight gain. We call these "overeating styles":

- Food Fretting
- Task Snacking
- Emotional Eating
- Fast Foodism
- Solo Dining
- Unappetizing Atmosphere
- Sensory Disregard

These overeating styles offer insights into what we were hoping to find out when we started searching for the way of eating that had led to normal weight for so long, and what we're doing differently today. The eating styles may seem subtle on the surface, but they're all−encompassing in that not only does each one influence weight, but we believe they all have a powerful impact on physical, emotional, spiritual, and social well−

being. Our findings clearly indicate that *the more we veer away from the way of eating that worked for humankind for millennia, the more likely we are to be overweight.* What's especially disconcerting is this: they represent the "new normal" way of eating for many of us.

Here's a closer look at these "new normal" eating styles:

1. Dieting and worrying about the "best" way to eat (food fretting)
2. Eating while doing other activities, such as driving or working (task snacking)
3. Turning to food to counteract negative feelings (emotional eating)
4. Consuming fast, processed food (fast foodism)
5. Eating alone (solo dining)
6. Eating while stressed (unappetizing *psychological* atmosphere), perhaps in your car (unappetizing *physical* atmosphere)
7. Eating quickly and not really tasting your food (sensory disregard)

Clearly, all seven overeating styles strongly diverge from the six perennial principles that served as eating guidelines in the past. Psychologist and obesity expert Kelly D. Brownell of the Rudd Center for Food Policy and Obesity at Yale University, might explain our findings as "modern food conditions and their mismatch with evolution,"[18] because the essence of our findings is that there's a huge disparity between what and how we eat today and what and how human beings ate and evolved for millennia. As a society, we have systematically moved away from the time–tested, integrative modes of eating and living that kept us slim for centuries. The way we ate and lived for thousands of years worked. The "new normal," the way we've been eating and living for the past few decades, doesn't.

Make Weight Loss Last

This is a book about losing weight and keeping it off—and accomplishing this by creating a pleasurable, positive, balanced relationship to food and eating . . . for life. In the chapters ahead, we'll introduce you to ten changes that have occurred during the last few decades that are making you fat, and ten solutions that nourish body, mind, and soul. Ultimately, what we're showing you is how to catch up with your culinary past so that you can claim your normal—weight heritage now.

What are the questions we often ask people who lose weight and keep it off? We want to know what they did to achieve such success—what they eat, or how much, or perhaps what their lifestyles are. For a long time, conventional wisdom told us that weight comes down to the calories—in/calories—out formula—that is, how much we eat and how much we exercise. Surely how much you eat and how much energy you use remain key players in the weight—loss puzzle. But in *Make Weight Loss Last*, we look beyond conventional wisdom by thinking of weight in terms of a *family* of eating behaviors and lifestyle choices. Unraveling *all* the elements we talk about throughout this book and identifying the ones that work for *you* is your best insurance for a lifetime of weight—loss success.

To get started, meet the eating styles and fill out our personalized "What's Your Overeating Style?" profile in Chapter 1. This quiz will reveal the degree to which you are practicing—or not—each overeating style. You'll discover how the *food choices* you make work together with the *eating behaviors* you typically practice to contribute to overeating and weight gain.

Once you find your trouble spots and the areas in which you can improve, the ensuing chapters will give you scientifically sound insights into each overeating style, along with the antidotes you can use to turn trouble areas into strengths. Throughout, you'll find personalized choices and actions you can use daily. These eating skills, tools, and insights are what you need to change the way you think about food, dieting, eating, and achieving and maintaining normal weight. The end result: you'll be able to turn your personal team of eating styles into a new relationship to food that empowers you to make weight loss last.

Beyond the Overeating Styles

In addition to the seven overeating styles and their solutions, we'll describe how three additional dynamics can cause you to pack on pounds. These, too, veer far from the way we ate and lived until recently: man—made chemicals in our meals, inadequate sleep, and too little exercise.

When most of us consider today's standard American diet (SAD), images of fast food, sugary beverages, and highly processed food "products" likely come to mind. Yet recent research has shown that there's more to our growing girth than too much fast food: a mud-dled brew of synthetic chemical compounds has made its way into our food and beverages and is playing havoc with our hormones—and, in turn, our weight. Chapter 9, "Quit Chemical Cuisine," sheds light on this relatively new saboteur of weight.

For millennia, humans awakened with the light of day and went to sleep when it got dark. During the twentieth century, 24/7 access to electricity made it possible for us to change our sleep cycle with the flip of a switch. Add a too-much-to-do, too-little-time-to-do-it lifestyle, and you have an equation for sleeping less and weighing more. Can a change in the number of hours you sleep each night make a difference in how much you weigh? What are the consequences of stepping away from the sleep cycle that sustained, reju-venated, and healed humans for so long? Chapter 10, "Sleep More, Weigh Less," addresses these questions.

Chapter 11, "Get Moving," offers insights into the weight-loss benefits of including more motion in your life. You'll find tools to help get yourself moving and a menu of movement options from which to choose.

Filled with practical guidelines that show you how to put our ten solutions into action each day, the final chapter gives you "Winning Weight Loss Strategies." There's a caveat, of course: success depends on *your* dedication and commitment to take action in ways that will work for you.

Make Weight Loss Last gives you the re-visioning and under-standing you need to redefine the role of food and eating in your life, so that you can "get back to the future" and make weight loss last. And it does more, for it aims at healing the split between today's state-of-the-art nutritional science and food's timeless place in the evolution of humankind. In this way, our book gives you the structure and the tools you need to nourish body, mind, and soul—and make weight loss last by finding true nourishment.

Chapter 1

What's Your Overeating Style?

The Make Weight Loss Last program, with its solutions to seven overeating styles, is unlike any eating plan you have ever followed in the past. It is not a quick–fix "diet." It is not about counting calories, figuring fat, or watching your weight. It's not low–carb or high–protein, nor is it a restrictive regimen. We're not suggesting the traditional, nonscientific approaches to eating and weight loss because, over the decades, we've learned that these either don't work or cannot be sustained. And the reason, we've discovered, is that they don't address the *underlying* reasons why most of us overeat.

In contrast, Make Weight Loss Last is effective as a strategy to lose weight and keep it off because it is the first comprehensive plan that gives you a way of eating and living that addresses many of the biological, psychological, spiritual, and social reasons you overeat. This program, then, is actually an expression of the ancient, original meaning of "diet" in the best sense of the word: it's a way of life and eating that can lead you naturally to weight loss and wellness.

Why do we describe this program as a way to live and not as a traditional diet? If your intention is to lose weight and you stay with our program, you'll likely succeed. At the same time, you will also be rewarded with more balanced emotions, spiritual well–being, and social connection. The multidimensional ways in which the solutions to the overeating styles heal are what we call "whole person nutrition," because you will discover not only optimal eating strategies for weight loss, but also how to make the most of your meals so that "all of you" will be nourished each time you eat. As you become more and more successful on this program, you will feel more and more fulfilled without overeating, at the same time experiencing both weight loss and "wellness living."

The point is this: throughout *Make Weight Loss Last*, we will show you how your relationship to food can be integrated into almost all aspects of your life, perhaps more so than any other activity. This has profound implications in terms of your well−being. Taking the time to appreciate food, eating with others, and slowing down to actu−ally focus on food—preparation, eating, even clean−up, not only can reduce stress and help you take charge of the hectic life many of us live but also can foster a deeper enjoyment of life.

Meet the Seven Overeating Styles

Have you thought much about your relationship to food? The com−plex of behaviors, feelings, and thoughts we bring to food are what comprise the seven overeating styles we've identified. If you're a "food fretter," for instance, you may diet a lot and judge food as "good" or "bad." Perhaps you're a "task snacker" who eats while you watch TV, work, or drive. Are you an "emotional eater" who binges when you're bored, anxious, or depressed? Is fast food, eaten alone and so quickly that you don't really taste it, your most−of−the time fare? Or do you typically relate to food with all—or none—of the overeating styles?

The seven overeating styles we discovered during our research on weight loss gave us new insights into the *reasons* so many of us overeat and gain weight, and what we can do about them.[1] We call these pat−terns of eating "styles" because they are sets of related behaviors that occur consistently over time. They are a unique expression of per−sonal style in terms of how you live or behave in relationship to food and food−related activities, from shopping for your food to eating it—even the atmosphere in which you dine.

Think about the eating styles this way. Every day you make a decision to style your hair in a manner that you believe is attractive, interesting, easy, or comfortable. Ultimately, your hairstyle reflects your taste and becomes typical of you; it becomes your personal style. When you're feeling good about your hair, you might say you're having a good hair day; when it's not looking its best, you may call it a bad hair day. As with good, bad, and in–between hair days, each of the seven overeating styles provides insight into the spectrum of your food–related behaviors. On one end of the continuum, you are eating optimally; at the other end, you are more likely to overeat and gain weight.

What does it mean to eat optimally? It means you take the time to nourish your body with a balanced intake of nutrients in fresh whole food (biological nutrition); you get pleasure from food so that you feel satisfied each time you eat (psychological nutrition); you connect to the life force in food (spiritual nutrition); and—because we're social beings—you thrive when you dine with others, sharing convivial conversation in pleasant surroundings (social nutrition).[2,3]

The more you distance yourself from these multidimensional facets of food (see the Introduction for more about the four facets of food), the more you're likely to be practicing one or more of the seven overeating styles—which we think leads to increased risk for becoming overweight or obese. We are excited to tell you about the overeating styles—in part because most of them have been over–looked by dieters, health professionals, and the diet industry, but also because our research has shown all seven to be statistically signifi–cant. Without a doubt, they are linked to overeating. Another way of looking at the overeating styles is this: they decode the many rea–sons so many of us overeat and gain weight. By knowing your own overeating styles, you're poised to practice the solutions we provide throughout the book and break the cycle of overeating and weight gain. Here's a brief introduction to get you started.

Food Fretting

Good food, bad food. Legal food, illegal food. Sinful food, pure food. The food fretting overeating style is overly concerned about and focused on food, projecting moral judgment onto what we and others eat. If you are often filled with thoughts about what you or anyone else should or shouldn't eat, traditional dieting, or the "right" way to eat, or if you tend to base your self–worth and that of others on what or how much is eaten, the food fretting style is a key contributor to your overeating.

Do you see yourself in any of the following examples of food fretting?

"I was good today," you may think when you've managed to avoid unhealthful foods, stick to your diet, and eat what you think you should.

"When my food cravings become powerful and I eat foods that are bad, I feel so guilty" is typical self-think for many food fretters.

"She should resist that sinful chocolate cake. Doesn't she have any willpower?" you might think as you watch someone eat what she "shouldn't."

Overcoming this eating style begins with recognizing such judgmental, fret-filled chatter about food and eating. Being honest with yourself will be challenging, since being critical and feeling anxious about food has become common in our culture. But the work you do to overcome this overeating style will be well worth the effort, because it will enable you to replace fret-filled self-think with empowering smart-think.

In Chapter 2, "Jettison Judgment," we'll reveal the pitfalls of food fretting and the judgmental dimension of eating. As you'll see, a key underlying element of this weight-inducing eating style is traditional dieting, then berating ourselves if we go off the diet. We will give you specific strategies for turning judgmental thoughts and actions into a whole person, nonjudgmental eating style so that you can appreciate food as a social, ceremonial, sensual pleasure—one that doesn't need to result in weight gain.

Task Snacking

Some call it "multitasking," the French call it "vagabond eating," and many in America think it's "normal." However it's perceived, if you often eat while working by yourself in front of your computer or while driving, watching TV, standing at the kitchen counter, shopping, or talking on the phone, it's likely that the "task snacking" eating style is increasing your likelihood of becoming overweight.

To counteract this overeating style, you'll discover how to rear—range your environment—both internally and externally. We'll show you how to work when you work, drive when you drive, and eat when you eat, rather than eating during other activities. You will find that making simple choices about eating mindfully can lead to big changes.

In Chapter 3, "Focus on Food," you'll discover how the behaviors linked to Task Snacking can contribute to weight gain. The anti—dote offered in the chapter will teach you how to break the cycle of merging eating with other activities. Eliminating task snacking com—pletely isn't necessarily the goal; instead, we'll give you easy actions that you can take right now to cut down on your food—related mul—titasking and, in turn, reduce your overeating—and weight.

Emotional Eating

Most of us are familiar with the phrase "emotional eating," turning to comfort food to soothe negative feelings (such as depression, anxiety, or loneliness) but also to enhance joyous, celebratory emotions (in response, let's say, to a wedding, birthday, or promotion). If you often eat to manage your feelings and to self—soothe—in other words, for reasons other than hunger—it's likely you're an emotional eater. Some health professionals describe this overeating style as "compul—sive overeating" or "food addiction." No matter what it's called, many of us turn to food to relieve emotional tension because it works. After all, doesn't eating certain foods serve as a distraction from emotions that may be making you uncomfortable?

It may not come as a surprise that our research pinpointed emo—tional eating as the strongest predictor of overeating—and, therefore, the key contributor to weight gain. What *is* groundbreaking are the specific emotions we've identified—the family of emotions—that are strongly linked with the likelihood that you'll overeat. Chapter 4, "Access Your Appetite," discusses the feelings that most strongly pre—dict overeating. We'll tell you about breakthrough brain—chemistry research that shows how turning to certain foods may mean you're self—medicating—which, in turn, may set off a binge in order to feel better. We shed light on the foods—and the specific nutrients in them—that can bust the blues, boost memory, cut carb cravings, and more. In essence, this chapter will give you the nutritional insights and tools you need to replace out−of−control emotional eating with the experience of a healthy appetite and food enjoyment.

Fast Foodism

A donut or sugary cereal for breakfast; a McDonald's double burger with fries for lunch; and a supersized pizza, perhaps placed casually on the dining table in its cardboard box, for dinner. Add several soft drinks throughout the day, and you have a profile of the fast−food cuisine that's typical for many Americans. Not surprisingly, this way of eating is strongly linked with overeating, overweight, and obe−sity—and it threatens more than your waistline.

As you'll discover, we qualify the solution with the phrase "as often as possible," to ensure that you don't interpret it as simply more dietary rules and regulations. Our intention is to help you think of what and how you eat as a spectrum rather than as all−or−nothing, black−or−white dietary dogma. To help you accomplish this, in Chapter 5, "Get Fresh," we show the link between fast foods and weight gain, and the added ingredients that keep you from achieving your health goals. We demystify optimal eating and offer practical tips, exercises, and strategies to help you achieve and maintain a healthy relationship to food, and well−being for a lifetime.

Solo Dining

Chapter 6, "Enjoy Food with Others," explains how dining alone can contribute to overeating and it shows you the "ingredients" and skills you need to create enjoyable dining experiences with others. To counteract the "solo dining" overeating style, we demonstrate how dining with others can be a balm for body, heart, and soul. You'll learn about the amazing healing possibilities of social dining that have been brought to light in scientific studies.

As your eating shifts from a "me" mentality to a "we" aware−ness—and, more and more, you share food and the dining experience with others—you'll be taking yet another step toward fulfillment and weight loss.

Unappetizing Atmosphere

You may find it surprising to learn that both the *psychological* and the *physical* atmospheres in which you eat can make a difference in whether or not you overeat and gain weight. Turning around the "unappetizing atmosphere" overeating style will quickly improve the quality of your life by enhancing how you feel both physically and emotionally. It may even improve your relationships—with others as well as with food.

The psychological and physical dining aesthetics of your life can contribute to satiety or lead to overeating. The psychological ele‐ ment refers to the emotions you experience within yourself and from others when you eat—feelings such as joy and happiness versus anger, fear, depression, and so on. The physical atmosphere includes your surroundings when you eat—at home, at the office, in restaurants, in your car, or at the homes of family and friends. Chapter 7, "Dine by Design," will give you a repository of strategies for accessing the healing power inherent in a relaxing, aesthetically pleasing, and wel‐ coming dining atmosphere.

Sensory Disregard

How often do you focus on the aromas, colors, or flavors of food? Do you "eat with your senses" by appreciating the presentation, "tasting" the textures, or being grateful for the life‐giving gift inherent in food? In our research, we found that those who ate the most actually enjoyed their food the least. Sensory disregard is a powerful predictor of overeating and weight gain, because if you're not enjoying your food—indeed, savoring it— you're likely to keep eating until you finally do feel a sense of satisfaction.

This may be the most overlooked aspect of overeating and ensuing weight gain. The problem is that most of us don't even know what it means to relate to food in this way, let alone have a clue about how to turn it into a way of eating that can make weight loss last. *Of all the overeating styles we've identified, sensory and spiritual disregard is associated with the largest number of food-related behaviors linked with overeating.*

Even if this eating style is unfamiliar territory for you, it's likely a major contributor to your overeating. If so, Chapter 8, "Feed the Senses," will give you insights into the price your mind, body, and waistline pay if you typically make and eat meals without flavoring them with sensory and spiritual ingredients. You'll discover how to turn meals into palate—pleasing adventures that nourish both body and soul, for when you eat from the heart, you enjoy your meals in a far more meaningful way.

What's Your Overeating Style?

How are you eating now? We've created a questionnaire to help you find out how much—or how little—each overeating style may be contributing to your overeating and weight gain. As you answer each question, you'll get a clearer idea about the many elements and behaviors that make up each eating style; at the same time, you'll raise your awareness about your own relationship to food. And when you tally your scores, you'll have created a personal eating style profile.

Completing the profile prior to reading the rest of this book will give you a baseline that you can use to measure improvements and changes in your eating styles. Consider the profile to be a lighthouse that helps you get your bearings, a guide for determining your eating style so that you can choose the direction that leads to the destination of your dreams. We mean this literally, because the concepts you'll be introduced to can be transformative. Here's your step—by—step guide to the profile.

Tally your scores. Complete each section of the following ques—tionnaire by checking the boxes that best represent your current eating style. Note that some sections have two parts. For these, score the top part by tallying all plus (+) numbers, the bottom part by adding up the minus (–) numbers. Then subtract the minus total from the plus total and enter the result at the bottom.

As you tally your scores, keep in mind that the numbers you come up with are more than just numbers. Negative numbers provide nuggets of knowledge about behaviors that lead to weight gain, while positive scores highlight actions linked to weight loss.

Interpret your scores. At the bottom of each style profile, you'll find a key that tells you whether your score ranks as "excellent," "good," "satisfactory," or "needs improvement." To discover your total score for all seven overeating styles, add the totals from the seven profiles; then read the interpretive section at the end.

FOOD FRETTING
Personal Profile

For each question, check the box in the column that best represents your "anxious eating" dynamic.

	Never	Rarely	Some-times	Usually	Almost Always	Always
	0	-1	-2	-3	-4	-5
1. I feel anxious about the "best" way to eat.	☐	☐	☐	☐	☐	☐
2. I feel "good" or righteous when I eat what I think I "should."	☐	☐	☐	☐	☐	☐
3. When I overeat, I feel:						
bad	☐	☐	☐	☐	☐	☐
guilty	☐	☐	☐	☐	☐	☐
gluttonous	☐	☐	☐	☐	☐	☐
4. I judge others by what they eat.	☐	☐	☐	☐	☐	☐
5. I try different diets.	☐	☐	☐	☐	☐	☐
6. I count calories, fat grams, etc.	☐	☐	☐	☐	☐	☐
7. I obsess about food.	☐	☐	☐	☐	☐	☐

Total Food Fretting Score: _____
Total

Food Fretting Scoring Key
  0 to -7   Excellent
 -8 to -14   Good
-15 to -21   Satisfactory
-22 or less   Needs Improvement

TASK-SNACKING
Personal Profile

For each question, check the box in the column that best represents your "task-snacking" dynamic.

	Never 0	Rarely -1	Some- times -2	Usually -3	Almost Always -4	Always -5
1. When I eat, I am...						
walking, rushing somewhere	☐	☐	☐	☐	☐	☐
at my desk at work	☐	☐	☐	☐	☐	☐
in my car	☐	☐	☐	☐	☐	☐
at my computer	☐	☐	☐	☐	☐	☐
talking on the phone	☐	☐	☐	☐	☐	☐
driving	☐	☐	☐	☐	☐	☐

Total Task-Snacking Score: _____

Total

Task-Snacking Scoring Key

0 to - 6	Excellent
-7 to -12	Good
-13 to - 17	Satisfactory
-18 or less	Needs Improvement

36

EMOTIONAL EATING
Personal Profile

For each question, check the box in the column that best represents your "emotional eating" dynamic.

	Never 0	Rarely +1	Some- times +2	Usually +3	Almost Always +4	Always +5
1. Before eating, I "check" my hunger level.	☐	☐	☐	☐	☐	☐
2. I eat only when I am hungry.	☐	☐	☐	☐	☐	☐

+ _____
Sub-total

	Never 0	Rarely -1	Some- times -2	Usually -3	Almost Always -4	Always -5
3. I overeat.	☐	☐	☐	☐	☐	☐
4. After eating, I feel stuffed.	☐	☐	☐	☐	☐	☐
5. I have food cravings.	☐	☐	☐	☐	☐	☐
6. I eat because I feel:						
depressed	☐	☐	☐	☐	☐	☐
sad	☐	☐	☐	☐	☐	☐
anxious	☐	☐	☐	☐	☐	☐
angry	☐	☐	☐	☐	☐	☐
frustrated	☐	☐	☐	☐	☐	☐
happy	☐	☐	☐	☐	☐	☐

− _____
Sub-total

Total Emotional Eating Score: (+) or (-) _____
Total

Emotional Eating Scoring Key
10 to -1   Excellent
-2 to -12   Good
-13 to -23   Satisfactory
-24 or less   Needs Improvement

FAST FOODISM
Personal Profile

For each question, check the box in the column that best represents your "fast food, fresh food" dynamic.

	Never 0	Rarely +1	Some- times +2	Usually +3	Almost Always +4	Always +5
1. I eat fresh:						
fruits	☐	☐	☐	☐	☐	☐
vegetables	☐	☐	☐	☐	☐	☐
whole grains	☐	☐	☐	☐	☐	☐
legumes	☐	☐	☐	☐	☐	☐
nuts	☐	☐	☐	☐	☐	☐
seeds (e.g., sunflower, flax)	☐	☐	☐	☐	☐	☐
2. I eat meals that are homemade.	☐	☐	☐	☐	☐	☐

+ _____
Sub-total

	Never 0	Rarely - 1	Some- times -2	Usually - 3	Almost Always - 4	Always - 5
3. I eat food that is:						
fast (such as McDonald's)	☐	☐	☐	☐	☐	☐
processed (canned, packaged)	☐	☐	☐	☐	☐	☐
prepared (deli, take-out)	☐	☐	☐	☐	☐	☐
sweet (donuts, muffins)	☐	☐	☐	☐	☐	☐
fried (potato chips, chicken)	☐	☐	☐	☐	☐	☐

− _____
Sub-total

Total Fast Food, Fresh Food Score: (+) or (-) _____
Total

Fast Food, Fresh Food Scoring Key

35 to 23	Excellent
22 to 11	Good
10 to -1	Satisfactory
-2 or less	Needs Improvement

SOLO DINING
Personal Profile

For each question, check every box in the column that best represents your "social fare" dynamic.

	Never 0	Rarely +1	Some-times +2	Usually +3	Almost Always +4	Always +5
1. I eat with:						
friends	☐	☐	☐	☐	☐	☐
family members	☐	☐	☐	☐	☐	☐
2. I eat at home at the dining table.	☐	☐	☐	☐	☐	☐
3. I enjoy preparing meals for friends.	☐	☐	☐	☐	☐	☐
4. I enjoy holiday feasts with others.	☐	☐	☐	☐	☐	☐
5. I celebrate special occasions with others with festive foods.	☐	☐	☐	☐	☐	☐
6. I prepare and share special meals for friends and family.	☐	☐	☐	☐	☐	☐
7. When eating alone, I often think about special people in my life, or memorable meals I've enjoyed with others.	☐	☐	☐	☐	☐	☐

+ _____
Sub-total

	Never 0	Rarely -1	Some-times -2	Usually -3	Almost Always -4	Always -5
8. I eat alone.	☐	☐	☐	☐	☐	☐
9. I plan "secret" overeating sessions.	☐	☐	☐	☐	☐	☐
10. I dine with others, then, afterward, binge by myself.	☐	☐	☐	☐	☐	☐
11. I stand at the counter while eating.	☐	☐	☐	☐	☐	☐

-- _____
Sub-total

Total Social Fare Score: (+) or (-) _____
Total

Social Fare Scoring Key

40 to 28	Excellent
27 to 16	Good
15 to 4	Satisfactory
3 or less	Needs Improvement

39

UNAPPETIZING ATMOSPHERE
Personal Profile

For each question, check the box in the column that best represents your "eating atmosphere" dynamic.

	Never 0	Rarely +1	Some- times +2	Usually +3	Almost Always +4	Always +5
1. The social atmosphere in which I prepare food is:						
serene	☐	☐	☐	☐	☐	☐
pleasing	☐	☐	☐	☐	☐	☐
fun	☐	☐	☐	☐	☐	☐
2. After eating, I feel:						
relaxed	☐	☐	☐	☐	☐	☐
calm	☐	☐	☐	☐	☐	☐
alert	☐	☐	☐	☐	☐	☐

+ _____
Sub-total

	Never 0	Rarely - 1	Some- times -2	Usually - 3	Almost Always - 4	Always - 5
3. The social atmosphere in which I prepare food is:						
hectic	☐	☐	☐	☐	☐	☐
tense	☐	☐	☐	☐	☐	☐

-- _____
Sub-total

Total Eating Atmosphere Score: (+) or (-) _____
Total

Eating Atmosphere Scoring Key

30 to 22	Excellent
21 to 14	Good
13 to 6	Satisfactory
5 or less	Needs Improvement

SENSORY DISREGARD
Personal Profile

For each question, check the box in the column that best represents your "sensory disregard" dynamic.

	Never 0	Rarely +1	Some-times +2	Usually +3	Almost Always +4	Always +5
1. I plan and prepare meals:						
with care	☐	☐	☐	☐	☐	☐
with appreciation	☐	☐	☐	☐	☐	☐
2. While dining, I consider my surroundings.	☐	☐	☐	☐	☐	☐
3. I express gratitude for food through prayer, blessings, heartfelt thankfulness.	☐	☐	☐	☐	☐	☐
4. I honor the mystery of life in food.	☐	☐	☐	☐	☐	☐
5. Before and during eating, I focus on the food's:						
color	☐	☐	☐	☐	☐	☐
aroma	☐	☐	☐	☐	☐	☐
portion size	☐	☐	☐	☐	☐	☐
flavor(s)	☐	☐	☐	☐	☐	☐
6. I "eat" with my senses, by:						
appreciating the presentation	☐	☐	☐	☐	☐	☐
tasting textures	☐	☐	☐	☐	☐	☐
savoring scents	☐	☐	☐	☐	☐	☐
7. I focus solely on food and the experience of dining.	☐	☐	☐	☐	☐	☐
8. I appreciate the "web" of humanity (farmers, grocers) surrounding food.	☐	☐	☐	☐	☐	☐
9. I consider the elements of nature that create food.	☐	☐	☐	☐	☐	☐
10. I eat with loving regard for food.	☐	☐	☐	☐	☐	☐
11. After eating, I:						
savor the moment	☐	☐	☐	☐	☐	☐
reflect on the meal	☐	☐	☐	☐	☐	☐

Total Sensory—Spiritual Nourishment Score: + _____
Total

Sensory Disregard—Spiritual Nourishment Scoring Key
72 to 90   Excellent
54 to 71   Good
53 to 36   Satisfactory
35 or less   Needs Improvement

Your Overeating Style Score

To find your Total Whole Person Nutrition Overeating Style Score:

1. Enter the **positive** scores for each of the seven eating styles in the "Positive Subtotals" column.

2. Enter the **negative** scores for each of the seven eating styles in the "Negative Subtotals" column.

3. For your total score, subtract the negative total from the positive total.

Eating Style	Positive Subtotals	Negative Subtotals
Food Fretting	_____	_____
Task Snacking	_____	_____
Emotional Eating	_____	_____
Fast Foodism	_____	_____
Solo Dining	_____	_____
Unappetizing Atmosphere	_____	_____
Sensory Disregard	_____	_____

Positive Total:_____ **Negative Total:**_____

TOTAL OVEREATING STYLE SCORE:_____

Evaluating Your Score

131 or more: Excellent. Congratulations! The "excellent" level is comparable to an A+. Your relationship with food is mostly satisfying and gratifying—you eat less and enjoy it more most of the time. Both what and how you eat are beneficial to your weight, your overall health, and your quality of life.

A score of "excellent" suggests that you are already practicing many of the solutions that make weight loss last. For still more bene−fits, look over your answers for each overeating style and target addi−tional changes you could make. Then turn to the chapters on the overeating styles for insights and tips on eating even more optimally.

130 to 55: Good. You're doing fairly well! The "good" level gives you a grade between A and B+. The foods you choose, how you eat, and with whom you eat are typically positive and beneficial. You eat optimally sometimes; when you're not able to—or choose not to—you let it go.

To improve your relationship to food and eating, look over your answers and decide whether there are changes you'd like to make to bring you closer to optimal eating. Then turn to the chapters on the overeating styles—particularly those to which you seem to have some resistance—for guidelines.

54 to −24: Satisfactory. Food and eating are often issues for you. The way you typically eat is comparable to a grade between B and C. You may have some confusion about what and how to eat optimally, or your overeating style hasn't been a priority so far. Your relation−ship to food and eating is fairly typical, which leaves lots of room for making beneficial changes.

A score of "satisfactory" suggests that you may find it challenging to practice many of the solutions we tell you about throughout *Make Weight Loss Last*. Look over your answers for each overeating style to target specific changes you'd like to make to lead you closer to optimal eating. Then turn to the chapters on the overeating styles for helpful suggestions.

−25 or less: Needs improvement. Your overall overeating style is far from optimal. Decide whether you want to take steps toward improving your relationship with food. To help you do this, first read the "Stages of Change" section in Chapter 2, "Jettison Judgment." Once you're clear about wanting to make changes, look over the questions in each section of the questionnaire for some quick and easy ways to get started.

A score of "needs improvement" suggests that you would benefit greatly by learning about, and then living, all the solutions we tell you about in *Make Weight Loss Last*. Look over your answers for each overeating style to target specific changes you'd like to make. Remember, small steps can lead to big benefits. Then turn to the chapters on the overeating styles to get started.

Haste Makes Waist

When we ask people in our workshops to share a memorable meal or dining experience, without fail they share stories that include the *solutions* to the overeating styles: (1) They anticipated the meal and ate it with pleasure, without judgment or anxiety; (2) they focused on the food and its flavor; (3) they enjoyed, indeed relished, the food, while being filled with positive feelings; (4) their meal was made with fresh ingredients; (5) they shared the experience with others; (6) they dined in pleasing surroundings; and (7) they appreciated the meal's sensory and spiritual ingredients. Their meal memories instinctively included all the elements of eating to make weight loss last: pleasure, mindfulness, feel−good emotions, fresh food, social connections, aesthetic awareness, and eating from the heart.

Whether the fare is simple or sublime, it's possible for you, too, to have memorable meals—and to manage your weight at the same time. How? By practicing and living the solutions to the seven overeating styles, so that body, mind, and soul are nourished each time you eat. Be aware, though, that what *you* contribute is as important, if not more so, than the insights and information we provide. There are three requisites for you to be successful: (1) a firm commitment to changing your approach to food and eating; (2) a willingness to take the necessary time to make beneficial changes; and (3) a commitment to a heartfelt regard for food and all food—related activities.

In the following chapters, we'll introduce you to researchers whose studies further our understanding of the mechanisms behind the various overeating styles. Each chapter gives insights and practical, pragmatic guidelines—the additional "ingredients" you need to reap the rewards of weight loss. In this way, you'll be empowered to overcome your own overeating styles and increase your chances of making weight loss last.

Chapter 2

Jettison Judgment

Not long ago, as I (co–author Deborah) chatted with a friend in front of a local supermarket while enjoying a piece of delicious dark chocolate, an acquaintance from the local health club walked by. "I see you," she said in response to what she perceived to be forbidden food. Knowing that we're knowledgeable about nutrition, this woman would often solicit an opinion about what and how much she should eat to lose weight. At other times, she'd walk up and—right after "Hello, Deborah"—give a detailed report on what she'd had for breakfast, lunch, and dinner the previous day, based on the diet du jour she was following. "What do you think of this diet?" she'd ask.

This same woman would occasionally take the liberty of describing a meal she'd eaten at a favorite restaurant. Had she made a "good" choice? Or not? And then there were the confessions about "sinful" desserts or "bad" carbs. She knew she "shouldn't eat these foods," but she missed them when she was "on a diet," so much so that she would often scarf down too much too quickly. "I know. I've completely blown my diet," would be her self–recriminating, guilt–laden lament. Then she would vow to "get back on track tomorrow."

This acquaintance is a textbook example of food fretting in action: dieting as a way of life; guilt, anxiety, and righteousness about the "best" way to eat; noticing what someone else is eating, then judging and even commenting on it; judging one's own food choices; eating by the numbers (calorie counting and weight watching, for example); and generally obsessing about food.

Although dieting, a judgmental attitude, and anxiety about food may not seem to have much in common, they share the distinguishing characteristics of a food fretter: feeling apprehensive about what food to eat, gluttonous when eating foods you think you shouldn't, and guilt when you go off your diet; and comparing yourself with others and then judging the differences. The key characteristic, though, is obsessing about food.

If you're a food fretter, you may also experience an alternating sense of righteousness or self−disdain—depending on how you're doing on your diet on a particular day. You tend to regard food with anxiety, and to judge what and how you eat as "good" or "bad" behaviors. You may even feel inadequate or envious when you see a thin person. The end result: much of your day−to−day thinking and ruminating is about food, "eating right," being thin—and often overeating.

Dieting Doldrums

If you think the food fretter's relationship to food, eating, dieting, and weight loss is normal—you're right. In America, 83 percent of college women diet no matter how much they weigh; two−thirds of Americans have tried some kind of weight loss diet; almost 50 per−cent of women are dieting on any given day, as is one in four men; and almost half the ten−year−old girls feel better about themselves when they're dieting.[1]

Dieting is a national obsession that is evident in the more than forty billion dollars we spend each year on dieting and related prod−ucts. Yet as our fixation on dieting increases, so, too, do our waistlines. More than 65 percent of adults over twenty−five are either over−weight or obese, up from 58 percent in 1983. And so are one in three children and adolescents.[2]

Regardless, millions of concerned Americans turn for help to diet books, surgery, or expensive spas. Still other gullible and desperate dieters succumb to quick−fix claims such as "Eat all you want and still lose weight" or "Melt away fat while you sleep." All the while, they remain oblivious to the secret of successful dieting: first and foremost, stop dieting.

Meet EDNOS

What's central to understanding the futility of food fretting and its family member, dieting, is that although it may be "normal," that doesn't translate into weight loss. More than 95 percent of dieters regain their lost weight in one to five years. Just as disheartening, 35 percent of "normal" dieters progress to pathological, obsessive dieting, while others develop full–blown eating disorders (EDs) such as anorexia nervosa, bulimia nervosa, or binge eating disorder (BED)—serious psychological conditions. What they have in common is that the sufferers are obsessed with food, diet, and often body image, which puts both their quality of life and their health at extreme risk.

EDNOS, the acronym for an "Eating Disorder Not Otherwise Specified," covers that gray area of disordered eating patterns that lies between optimal, healthful eating and clinical eating disorders. People with an EDNOS may diet chronically, focus on weight constantly, or binge occasionally. In other words, food and eating are a major source of stress for people with EDNOS. And this means they are food fret–ters and at risk for overeating and weight gain.

I (co–author Deborah) remember as a child watching my mother jump into the dieting ditch. She and a few of her friends had just returned from their first Weight Watchers meeting, in the early days of Weight Watchers when founder Jean Nidetch was at the helm. Sitting at our kitchen table, I watched as my mother and her friends displayed the little tabletop food scales they would use to weigh their food. On the surface, the dieting ritual they had just learned and were practicing with food from the fridge seemed like harmless fun and an opportunity to socialize. But now, when I revisit the scene from the perspective of an adult and a researcher who knows about food obsession and dieting, I perceive that evening as the start of my mother's formalized, ritualized food fretting. She told me that as a young adult, she often tried to will herself to abstain from foods she enjoyed so that she could "keep her figure." Now, as an adult and the mother of two children, watching her weight by dieting, weighing, and counting had become a way of life.

My mother's experience is typical of dieters: she entered the world of food fretting gradually, with high expectations of success—

losing weight and maintaining a healthy weight. But because she didn't know that the seemingly simple, seemingly achievable vision she was pursuing was really radical and difficult, she struggled with the battle of the bulge for years.

The Dieting Dilemma

Recent scientific discoveries that weren't available to my mother's generation have a lot to tell us about why dieting and obsessing about food doesn't work—and what you can do to escape, permanently, from the dieting gulag in which many of us are confined.

When we discovered the seven overeating styles that lead to over–weight and obesity, we realized that losing weight and keeping it off is based on a complex matrix of food– and eating–based thoughts, behaviors, and feelings. The results you want—enjoying food and eating as a way of life that leads naturally to weight loss and physical health, emotional well–being, spiritual sustenance, and social sup–port—may call for making long–term changes not only to what and how much you eat, but especially to why and how you eat.

As a first step toward getting where you want to be, consider three questions that lie at the heart of getting off the food–fretting tread–mill of dieting and obsessing about food. Are your weight goals and expectations realistic? Is there a "best" (regimented) diet that works for the long term? Are you really ready to make the changes necessary to lose weight, or do you just think (and hope) you are?

Reframing Successful Dieting

Most diet and weight–loss programs ask you to set a "goal weight," establishing the number of pounds you need to lose to achieve a tar–geted weight. If you buy into this popular norm, you may be setting yourself up for failure. Consider novel research on goal weight and how it sabotages success that was conducted by obesity researcher Gary D. Foster in the late 1990s. Foster, director for the Center for Obesity Research and Education at Temple University, wanted to explore why so many of us fail at dieting. To find out, he and his team asked sixty obese women to identify how many pounds they would need to lose to achieve what they considered their "dream" weight, "happy" weight, "acceptable" weight, and "disappointed" weight. At the end of the forty–eight weeks of the weight–loss program, almost half hadn't achieved even their "disappointed" weight. When the researchers replicated the study with 154 overweight people, this time including men, again those least successful at losing weight were the most obese with the most unrealistic weight–loss "dream" goals.[3]

If we didn't know that obsessing about weight contributes to failure, we might think that the dieters didn't have the willpower to reach their goal weight. We might imagine that the diet they followed was too hard and strict, that the dieters weren't really committed to losing weight, or perhaps that there were biological or genetic reasons for their failure. But the food–fretting mentality inherent in targeting a goal weight suggests something quite different. It tells us that obsessing about a particular number (how much you'd like to weigh) isn't an effective or realistic (or pleasant) way to lose weight. It simply doesn't work. And not only doesn't it work, but with such high dropout rates, there seems to be something that's actually counterproductive about setting a goal weight.

A more recent comprehensive national study led by investigator Riccardo Dalle Grave, an obesity researcher from Italy, supports Foster's findings and the futility of food fretting as an effective way to lose weight. When Dalle Grave and his colleagues assessed the weight–loss expectations of 1,785 obese people seeking treatment at twenty–three medical centers, they discovered that the dropouts had more pounds to lose to achieve their "dream" weight compared with the continuers who finished the study. In fact, the strongest predictor that people would drop out of the study was the degree to which their weight–loss expectations were unrealistic.[4]

Both Foster and Dalle Grave interpreted their goal weight studies in a similar way: because unrealistic weight–loss expectations increase the likelihood that an overweight person will give up, more modest weight–loss goals may be a more realistic way to lose weight. But stopping the food fretting and reframing what constitutes successful weight loss has even larger implications, because even modest weight loss can bring big health benefits.

There are three interesting insights to be gained from these studies. The first is that unrealistic expectations and goals about weight loss lead to disappointment and giving up. And feeling that your efforts are futile makes it likely that you will, indeed, go off your diet and fail to lose weight. A second insight is that the goal weights chosen by the obese participants in the studies were three times as great as the actual weight they lost. The message we can take away from this is that it would be wise to reduce the initial goal, perhaps by as much as two–thirds, and then set another modest goal weight after the initial weight–loss phase.

The third insight has to do with how you think of yourself. Since participants' body images and self–esteem were tied to how much weight they wanted to lose (the lower the self–image, the more extreme and unrealistic the goal weight), it would be smart to reverse the formula: work on esteem and body image to reduce unrealistic expectations and increase the likelihood of success.

If you suffer from one or more medical problems related directly to your weight, knowing that you can achieve big benefits with just a small amount of weight loss is powerful news. Lose just ten pounds and your triglyceride levels (a risk factor for heart disease) can drop as much as 34 percent, your total cholesterol can decrease 16 per–cent, LDL (bad) cholesterol can decrease 12 percent, and HDL (good) cholesterol can increase 18 percent. If you have high blood pressure or diabetes, you may be able to reduce or discontinue medications with a loss of only 5 to 10 percent of your current weight. And if degenerative joint disease such as osteoarthritis is a problem for you, every 2.2 pounds of weight lost reduces the stress on each knee by approximately five pounds per square inch. This could translate into delaying or negating the need for knee surgery.[5]

Small changes can bring big benefits. Even modest but sustained weight loss, without targeting an ideal body weight, can improve many weight–related ailments and your overall health and well–being. And you're likely to look better and to feel better about yourself.

As simple as it sounds, shifting your thinking from reaching an ideal weight to establishing reasonable expectations is a dramatic paradigm shift, according to Foster. Reframing weight–loss success calls for a major change in the diet—think that permeates our culture. But the health rewards of losing even a modest amount of weight are great. And when you stop dieting and reframe your idea of successful weight loss, you'll experience less stress around food, eating, and your weight, and more peace of mind.

Unrealistic weight—loss goals may be a key food—fretting culprit that keeps you from attempting to lose weight, or actually losing it, and feeling good about yourself. But if changing the way you think about weight—loss success is an important piece of the weight—loss puzzle, would it be helpful if you also changed the way you think about diets themselves—especially if you knew that they can destroy the likelihood that you'll lose weight and keep it off?

Diet More, Weigh More

The strongest food—fretting predictor that you'll overeat and gain weight is traditional dieting. If you live your life on a diet and restrict your calories with the intention of losing weight, you're actually put—ting yourself at risk for gaining weight.

Earlier in this chapter, we mentioned that about 95 percent of those who lose weight on a traditional diet gain it back. If you've followed this track, it's likely you lost some weight while you were on the diet; after all, if you restrict your calories you will lose weight. But you're also likely to lose a lot more: muscle mass and a speedy metabolism. This is of special concern, because if your muscles and your metabolism (the rate at which your body processes food) are in good shape, it's easier to lose weight and keep it off. But cut calo—ries, and both your muscles and your metabolism weaken, sabotaging weight loss. Here's why.

Muscles. The amount of energy (calories from food) your body needs each day is based on your basal metabolic rate as well as your daily physical activity. For most or us, this equals 1,500 to 2,500 calo—ries per day. Reduce your daily caloric intake to below what your body needs (in other words, go on a diet) to, say, 1,200 calories, and your body goes into survival mode. After all, it doesn't know you're a woman on a calorie—restricted diet whose goal is to fit into a size

6; no, your body thinks it's starving. To keep this from happening—especially if you aren't exercising or doing weight−resistance exercises—it turns to your muscle tissue and breaks it down for energy. And once you lose muscle mass, your body will need even fewer calories than it did prior to dieting; in other words, you'll need to consume even less food to lose weight or keep it off.

There's more bad news. Because your muscle mass is providing the energy you need, even if you lose twenty−five pounds on your low−calorie diet, you'll be losing muscle and fat in equal amounts. *And your body will actually become more efficient at storing fat by slowing down your metabolism.*

Metabolism. When your metabolism is performing optimally, your body efficiently burns the calories from your food. If you don't eat enough food, though, your metabolism slows down and you don't burn calories as quickly. As you continue to starve yourself (at least, this is what your body thinks you're doing), your metabolism burns food calories more slowly. When you stop your restrictive diet, your metabolism stays slow, making it easier to gain the weight back even faster, even if you still cut calories and eat less than before you decided to diet.

In other words, *low-calorie diets make your body more efficient at storing fat—not losing it—and they slow down your metabolism, making it harder—not easier—for you to lose weight.*

There's another catch−22 to cutting calories: you actually train your mind to obsess about food. Here's why. First you're told, or you decide, to visualize how you want to look at your "ideal" weight. Some diet experts even suggest that you put a picture of a person at your "perfect" visualized weight on your refrigerator to serve as a reminder to stay on your diet. Then there are the food lists, exchanges, and points. Is this food permitted or not? Is it low carb or high fat? Whichever way you turn the grocery cart, it's geared to keep you thinking and thinking and thinking about food—in other words, obsessing about it. Add the fact that you're being told what and how much you can eat, and you're setting yourself up for a food mutiny!

Ergo, you break your diet and eat the foods you've been craving—and as much of them as you let your craving drive you to eat.

The Four Diets Study

A recent research project verifying that diets aren't the path to losing weight was motivated by the scarcity of studies on the topic. To find out whether popular diet plans (Atkins, Zone, Weight Watchers, and Ornish) actually work—whether there is a "best" diet that health practitioners can recommend for weight loss and reduced risk of heart disease—researchers randomly assigned 160 overweight or obese adults aged twenty–two to seventy–two to one of the four popular diets. During the first two months, both a doctor and a dieti–tian trained participants. Then they were on their own for ten more months, until the weigh–in after a year of dieting.

When the results were tallied, the researchers discovered that while each diet significantly lowered bad cholesterol and increased good cholesterol, the dropout rate was substantial for all four: 53 per–cent for Atkins, 50 percent for Ornish, and 35 percent for Zone and Weight Watchers. And even though there was a slight average weight loss (4.6 to 7.3 pounds) after one year for those who managed to stay on one of the diets, the number of pounds lost didn't register as being statistically significant. In short, no diet was better than another for weight loss; indeed, no study participants lost significant amounts of weight—regardless of the diet.

When we lecture about whole person nutrition and the seven overeating styles, the question we're asked most frequently is about the diet du jour. Many want to know which diet is best. Is it the Zone? Eat Right 4 Your Type? What do we think about Ornish (high carbohydrate/low fat) versus Atkins (high protein/high fat)? Which do we choose?

The simple answer is that we *don't* choose, because we know that diets don't work and that, instead, they lead to a sense of failure and self–esteem problems. Clearly, we're asking the wrong question ("What's the best diet?"), so we're getting the disappointing answer of ongoing weight gain. This may seem obvious, but it isn't. "I would suspect that most of the popular diet books in the bookstore are likely to produce weight loss if you follow the plan closely, since almost all plans are similar to the diets we studied, or to a cross between two of them," Michael L. Dansinger, MD, leader of the study, told WebMD. "Date the diets until you can find a life partner. The best way is to try a number of them."[6]

As Dansinger suggests, all weight−loss diets work if dieters stick with them—but most don't, for the reasons reviewed throughout this chapter. The four−diets study confirms that all diets are challenging to stay with, even under quality supervision (doctors and dietitians), and that for most people diets aren't the answer for long−term weight loss.

Two other aspects of the study also caught our attention. We find it interesting that the Atkins, Zone, Weight Watchers, and Ornish diets chosen for the study have a lot in common: as with all diets, they omit the junk food and fast food that typically contribute to weight gain. What you're *not* eating plays a big part in determining whether or not you lose weight and keep it off. The other aspect of the study we find intriguing is its focus on each diet's proportion of macro−nutrients (carbohydrates, fat, and protein) and, to a lesser degree, micro−nutrients (such as vitamins and minerals). The nutrient composition of food plays an important role in preventing, man− aging, or reversing a health condition such as heart disease, diabetes, and depression. For instance, if you have heart disease or high cho− lesterol, the nutrient composition of the Ornish diet is optimal for reversal. But a diet's macro− and micro−nutrient balance isn't the key to optimizing weight loss; balancing energy input (food) and output (physical activity) is.

Are You Really Ready to Lose Weight?

Two decades ago, psychologists James Prochaska and Carlo DiClemente developed a model for how people change their lifestyle habits that was exceptional in three important ways. First, their model is sup− ported by scientific studies. Secondly, their ideas are unique in that they reframe successful lifestyle change that "sticks" as a step−by−step process, one that requires an experiential shift in a person's attitude, perception, and way of being. Without graduating through succes− sive steps (five stages of change), individuals are more likely to fail to make lasting change. And finally, their model tells us that making long—term changes often involves setbacks, but that with repeated efforts the chances for success increase. In other words, change—such as losing weight—is not a black—or—white, all—or—nothing decision. Prochaska and DiClemente posit that to achieve lasting change, it's quite normal that people need to make more than one attempt.[7]

Today, the psychologists' model is a cornerstone of the Trans—theoretical Model of Change used by many health professionals and in dozens of programs that help people with behavioral addictions as well as substance abuse and addictions to drugs, cigarettes, and alcohol.

Although overeating and related disorders may feel like addic—tions to those who struggle with them, they technically aren't classed as such because the chemical process linked to addictive behavior is different from the chemical changes that occur in your brain when you eat different foods (for more about how food affects mood, see Chapter 4, "Access Your Appetite"). Rather, the food you eat may be considered a "substance" that creates chemical changes in the brain, which in turn influence feelings. Those with EDNOS, who abuse food (and their bodies), are likely to have a substance abuse problem, not an addiction (see the Introduction for more about food addic—tion). Food—related behaviors are considered to be deeply instilled habits that, for most of us, are hard to change—unless you find out where you are in the stages of change model and then progress through each stage.

Stages of Change

The stages of change model gives us insights about how to change and specific strategies for how you can best help yourself in your effort to become a "successful loser." The mistake most of us make when we think of losing weight by "going on a diet" is being igno—rant about where we are in the cycle. Once you know which stage you're in, you can rationally and thoughtfully progress to the next stage. By not jumping ahead to a stage for which you may not be ready (such as dieting), you lower the odds of slipping back into old eating habits.

When Prochaska and DiClemente did their initial study and identified the five stages of change, it was with 872 people who were hoping to change their smoking habits. The five stages they identified are precontemplation, contemplation, preparation, action, and maintenance; people who revert to precontemplation, contemplation, or preparation during their efforts to change are said to be in relapse stage.

Are you really ready to lose weight, or do you just want to? Spend time with the stages and you'll know the answer. Take the time to identify the stage you're in right now. You'll know if and when you are ready to change your food fretting when you understand the stage you're in and stay with that stage until you're truly, deep-down ready to move on to the contemplation stage or the action stage. Empowered by these self-insights, you'll be poised to turn the defeatism of traditional dieting upside down.

Precontemplation. This is a kind of precursor to the four other, more formal stages that empower you to change your food choices, eating behaviors, and weight. You're in the precontemplation stage If you're not yet interested in changing your food and eating habits ("This is the way I am; I'm big-boned"), if you're not concerned about being overweight ("Most Americans are overweight; I fit right in"), or if you don't recognize that you have a problem with food or weight ("It's society's problem, not mine"). You may also be ignorant of health risks linked with overweight or obesity and, instead, blame your weight on biology, metabolism, or genes inherited from your parents. You're not too open to advice, and you're not yet contemplating change.

Contemplation. If you're thinking about changing what and how you eat, and you're kind of easing into it—perhaps you'll get to it tomorrow or sometime in the next few months—you are in the contemplation stage. At this stage, you may have some ambivalence, because considering a change in lifelong food habits can be a life-altering decision. As you progress through contemplation, you will come to a decision about your next step.

Preparation. If you're in this stage, you've decided to make a change; you've shifted from "I ought to" to "I'm going to." Making changes in your food choices and overeating styles is just around the corner; you plan to do it within the next month. To prepare for success when you make your shift into action, you first weigh the pros and cons. What's the downside to what and how you're currently eating? What are the benefits you'll receive by changing your relationship to food? What's working well for you? What exactly needs to change? You're getting in touch with the downside of food fretting; at the same time, you're considering, organizing, and planning the benefits of de–food fretting. After you've thought through the pros and cons, it's time to create your plan of action.

Action. During the preparation stage, you identified obstacles to making changes as well as strengths you bring with you along the journey. You have entered the action stage when you've prepared yourself for change and created specific steps. Now you're motivated and ready to implement the plan of action you've been thinking about for the past weeks or months. Not only are you clear about what you want to achieve and how you're going to go about it, but you're actually doing it and being it.

Maintenance. Maintaining optimal food choices, eating behaviors, and weight loss calls for progressing through the previous stages until they become habitual. Keep in mind that it typically takes weeks to change a habit (twelve weeks is a guesstimate), and to achieve lasting change. This may be a good time to weigh the benefits and obstacles you identified in the preparation stage, and to make changes accordingly.

Relapse. The stages of change aren't an all–or–none proposition (unlike most diets); rather, they're a process, guidelines for transitioning from food fretting and yo–yo dieting to lasting change. Realize that it's common to return to what's familiar and comfortable, even though it may not be what you want or what's good for you. Realize that many of us will relapse and return to prior eating habits and food choices for a short or long time. This isn't the time to get discouraged and give up.

Instead, go back over the stages and plan how to overcome the obstacle that got in your way; when you've done this, return to the action stage. Be compassionate with yourself, and repeat each of the stages until the action stage becomes second nature.[8]

De–Food Fretting Strategies

There's a lot more you can do to de–food fret and overcome your food–related anxieties, self–recrimination, judgment, and guilt. Here's a look at what it takes to transcend the cycle of dieting and obsessing about food and weight.

Don't diet. More and more research is linking traditional dieting with increased risk of weight gain. Consider "dieting" in the best sense of the word. The word "diet" comes from the Old French *diete* or Greek *diaeta*, meaning "mode of life." Hippocrates, the father of modern medicine, used *diet* as a "prescribed mode of life," which eventually evolved into meaning "prescribed regime of food."[9] We're suggesting that you diet as an expression of the ancient meaning of the word, as a way of life: that you relate to eating as a social, cer–emonial, and sensual delight, and to food as a gift that enhances your physical, emotional, spiritual, and social well–being.

Stop counting calories. Traditional diets that ask you to restrict calories and to eat by the numbers (calories, fat grams, and so on) are no longer appropriate. To lose weight, you don't need more numbers; you need other ways of relating to food so that each time you eat you have an enjoyable experience that nourishes your entire being. Instead of staying lost in a maze of measurements, nutrients, and numbers, focus on fresh foods, flavors, the profound pleasure of eating, and the delight you take in dining with others.

Halt judgment. In 1987, co–author Deborah's father died abruptly of a heart attack; her mother also died of heart disease—congestive heart failure. Having worked as the nutritionist with Dean Ornish on his first clinical trial for reversing heart disease and later as the director of nutrition on a similar research project in Europe, she knew a lot about nutrition, lifestyle, and health, yet still couldn't seem to find the "right" or "best" way to help her parents. "I knew my parents understood the heart—healthy dietary and other lifestyle information I'd given them, but in retrospect I realize that the underlying message I was giving was, 'You *should* be eating differently. You *should* stop eating familiar and comfortable foods. You *should* assess and analyze what you're eating.'"

Should. It simply doesn't work—for you or for others. How did so many of us learn to judge both ourselves and others' food choices and eating habits? In the late 1800s, Puritan values still predominated in America, which meant that food was often perceived as sinful, or as good and bad; we projected moral values onto food—and still do. Instead, we need to view food, eating, and the experience of dining as a celebration of life.

Give up guilt-tripping. Guilt and its relatives—self—reproach, shame, remorse, and blame—are part of a food fretter's relationship to food. It's all about what is "right" and what is "wrong." Eat some—thing "wrong" that isn't on your diet, that you "shouldn't," that tastes "sinful," and—if you're a food fretter—you're likely to respond with guilt. The dictionary tells us that to feel guilty is to feel remorse about having done something wrong. The link between guilt and wrong—doing has roots in the word's Old English meaning: "crime."[9] Is eating food you "shouldn't" eat a crime? Or, as with the food—fretter feeling of judgment, when you feel guilt over something you ate (or want to eat), are you projecting a moral value onto the food and in the process making yourself miserable?

Consider this: guilt isn't a real feeling. At its core lies the belief you've done something wrong, and now you must suffer for it. To break that conviction and get the upper hand over guilt, change what you choose to believe. Replace guilt—laden thoughts with a positive picture. Realize that you can't undo what was done . . . and simply accept it. Finally, forgive yourself, for forgiveness is a necessity in any relationship—including the one you have with food.

Cease obsessing. If you're fixated on and preoccupied with food–related thoughts, feelings, and behaviors, if you think or worry about food or weight constantly and compulsively, you are obsessing. The way out is to step from the shade in which you're living, into the sunshine. Meditation can help you do this.

Meditation and Meals

A conversation in a café with a new acquaintance first brought home the power of meditation as a way to let go of food fretting and replace it with naturally occurring weight loss. Midway through the get–together, she said she had lost twenty pounds as a side effect of meditating regularly. Accessing the wisdom within yourself through regular meditation is one path you can take to de–food fret and create a more balanced relationship to food, eating, and your weight.

Meditation, with its myriad variations, has been espoused as a spiritual discipline by religions, philosophies, and traditions for thou–sands of years. In the East, yogis say it leads to a super–conscious state that emerges from the cessation of thought. Taoists tell us it leads to a sense of harmony with all things and a return to the depths of the self, while proponents of Zen perceive meditation as a path to sudden illumination. In the West, it is often linked with the mystical and monastic. Judaism's mystical Kabbalah teaching turns to meditation to carry consciousness through various "gateways," early Christian monks and saints used it as a stringent contemplative process to achieve spiritual exaltation, and Islam's spiritual Sufis interpret it as a way to suffuse their minds, hearts, and souls with "higher things."

The ancient tradition of meditation comes from the Latin *meditari*, meaning deep, continued reflection. Over the millennia, many types have evolved. For instance, *apophatic* meditation is designed to empty the mind by eliminating thoughts from consciousness, while the *cataphatic* focus is on holding a specific image, idea, or word in the mind's eye, allowing emotions to manifest themselves.

During the past decades, many scientific studies have verified the ways in which meditation can heal body, mind, and soul. Vipassana meditation, an ancient practice from India that was rediscovered by Gotama Buddha more than 2,500 years ago, is an especially pow–

erful technique for food fretters. With its focus on self−transformation through self−observation, it is designed to dissolve chaotic, drifting thoughts that sabotage well−being and instead to bring balance and peace of mind. Using the same concept, we created a self−guided technique that we call "food−friendly meditation." We designed it as a meditation for food fretters who are often obsessive about food and eating, and whose thoughts are filled with anxiety and judgment about food, eating, and weight. It can be a powerful tool, for meditation can change both conscious and unconscious food−related behaviors.

The Food-Friendly Meditation

Before beginning our step−by−step food−friendly meditation, look over the "What's Your Overeating Style?" profile in Chapter 1 to identify the elements of food fretting with which you have the most trouble. Then, with each inhalation, imagine how each element makes you feel; with each exhalation, imagine a non−food fretting scenario. For instance:

• As you inhale, imagine how you feel when you are "on a diet"; exhaling, envision yourself eating tasty fresh food in a relaxed frame of mind.

• As you inhale, recall the guilt you feel after eating food you "shouldn't"; exhaling, delight in the flavor of a favorite food, without judgment.

• As you inhale, conjure up the image of an obese person eating in a restaurant; exhaling, feel compassion for the person.

To obtain the full benefit of the meditation, practice the fol−lowing steps for fifteen to thirty minutes each day. When your mind wanders, gently bring your attention back to the imagery.

1. Set aside some time when you will not be disturbed. Choose a comfortable place to sit, and sit in a comfortable upright position, with relaxed shoulders.
2. Close your eyes.
3. Position your head so it is comfortably balanced between your shoulders.
4. Inhale deeply, pause for two seconds, then exhale deeply. Do this three times.
5. As you inhale, say to yourself, "I know that I am breathing in."
6. As you exhale, say to yourself, "I know that I am breathing out."
7. Identify an element of food fretting that is problematic for you, such as dieting, guilt, or judgment.
8. Inhale the problematic *situation*; exhale the *solution*.

The food–friendly meditation gives you the skills you need to let food–fretting thoughts emerge—to simply observe the thoughts and behaviors—and then to let them go. Replace the thoughts you release with positive emotions such as acceptance, joy, pleasure, and compassion.

Staying focused, mindful, and in the moment is challenging; it's normal for our thoughts to wander. Given this tendency, realize that meditation is a lifetime process. When and if you find your mind wandering, bring your thoughts back to the meditation. Your intention is to stay with the meditation as long as possible and not to perceive it as something you have to do "perfectly."

Jettison Judgment

To eat—and live—optimally, consider that food is more than an amalgam of nutrients and calories leading to weight loss—or gain. Along with healing you physically, it can improve your mood, satisfy your soul, and connect you to others and to the mystery of life. If you're often filled with food fretting and thoughts of dieting, calorie–counting, and anxious overeating, here's the antidote:

Food Fretting Rx: Perceive food and the experience of eating as a social, ceremonial, sensual pleasure.

In other words, replace food fretting with the experience of enjoying food, and appreciate eating as one of life's pleasures. Use the insights and practical strategies in this chapter to turn your food fretting into a positive relationship to food and eating.

Chapter 3

Focus on Food

Some call it "multitasking"; the French call it "vagabond eating." In America, it's a growing trend. Whatever form it takes—eating a meal or snacking mindlessly while working in front of your computer, driving, watching TV, shopping with a friend, or talking on the phone—the task snacking overeating style puts you at risk for becoming overweight. Have you ever meandered through the mall while munching? If so, you're task snacking. Do you watch TV, flip through a magazine, or study while eating? These are more task-snacking behaviors. As a matter of fact, doing other things while you're eating is so common in our culture, it's become normal.

Consider "car cuisine," the growing tendency for drivers to eat in their cars at drive-through restaurants or while driving. As Americans eat more and more meals in their cars, food makers have accommodated them with what they call "cup-holder cuisine": finger-friendly foods and compact "meals" that are drop-free and glop-free. Examples include cereal bars made with dry milk; salad-in-a-cup and pancake-like breakfast sandwiches with the "yummy taste of maple syrup baked right in" (available at McDonald's); squeeze tubes containing yogurt; and drinkable soups that can be sipped from a cup. Some experts say that almost 20 percent of us consume such "meals" in cars. The "dashboard dining" trend is so entrenched that Honda provides a pop-up table in the console and Saab sells models with refrigerated glove boxes.[1]

Not only do most of us not pay much attention to where we're eating and what we're doing while we're eating, we also don't believe that these two factors have anything to do with our weight. But they do.

A Tale of Two Task Snackers

We vividly remember the moment we realized we were task snackers. We were at Heinrich–Heine, a medical university in Dusseldorf, Germany, where we'd been invited to do research on lifestyle (diet, stress management, exercise, and group support) and heart disease. After several months, when we'd become good friends with some colleagues, we heard a knock on our office door around lunchtime. "We're going to the cafeteria for lunch," said Siegfried. "Would you like to join us?" We stopped clicking away at our computers mid–word, put our homemade sandwiches away, gathered our coats, and walked through the wintry campus with three coworkers to the building that housed the cafeteria.

In place of sitting at our desk and working at our computers while eating our sandwiches, we were greeted by students' energetic conversations as they waited in line to choose their food. After our leisurely lunch, convivial conversation, and another chance to walk and talk in the fresh, crisp air, we all returned to work. We would repeat this welcome ritual with our friends many times during the two years we worked in Europe.

Upon reflection, we can't help but think how atypical such a social scenario has become for many Americans. Don't most of us munch mindlessly while working at our desks? One of the first studies to demonstrate the link between eating at your desk (a classic task–snacking behavior) and increased risk of weight gain was done by the American Dietetic Association, which cosponsored a survey with ConAgra Foods. When they polled 1,024 full–time employees who worked at desks, they discovered that most ate while working: 67 percent ate lunch, 61 percent nibbled munchies, and 37 percent ate breakfast. An additional 10 percent of men and 7 percent of women eating their dinners at their desks, continuing the habit of task snacking into the evening hours.

How might desktop dining translate into an increased risk for piling on pounds? Eating at your desk while working means you're likely to consume more food than you realize, suggests David Grotto of the American Dietetic Association.[2] Along with overeating, staying put also means you're moving less and therefore burning fewer calo–

ries than more motion–conscious coworkers. Not surprisingly, this can lead to the tired but true formula for weight gain: eating more and moving less.

"That's exactly what happened to me," exclaimed a physician friend of ours when we told him about the link between desktop dining and weight gain. "Because I was on deadline to complete my fifth book, I ate breakfast, lunch, and dinner while working at my computer, between seeing patients," he clarified. "During this time, my wife took over my job of walking our dog each day. After nine months, I finished the manuscript; at the same time, I was surprised to discover I had gained almost twenty pounds. This had never happened to me before." Our health–savvy friend said it took almost a year to get back to his normal weight.

Anatomy of Task Snacking

It's obvious that if you're a task–snacking couch or mouse potato, it's likely you're not moving much. And this means that, like our friend who put on twenty pounds while working on his book, lack of exercise is a key contributor to weight gain (more about this in Chapter 11, "Get Moving"). But how, specifically, might task snacking work against your waistline when you eat while working, munch while watching TV, or snack while driving? How is eating in a not–too–conscious, not–too–mindful way a recipe for weight gain?

Because the brain can attend to only one topic at a time, when you do multiple tasks simultaneously, it constantly shifts its attention. If you were to undergo a PET scan—Positron Emission Tomography, a powerful, noninvasive imaging technique that accurately images the cellular function of the human body—while task snacking, it would show lights blinking on and off in areas of the brain associated with the various tasks you're undertaking. When you eat while the mind isn't focused on your food, the digestive process is impaired, making food not nearly as nutritious as it could be. In turn, this can trigger hunger and the drive to eat more so that you'll feel satisfied via the nutrients your mind and your body need for optimal health—nutrients that you're not metabolizing. Thus task snacking can create a vicious cycle of poor digestion, inadequate nutrition, and overeating to try to get the vitamins and minerals you're not metabolizing.

Task snacking works on yet another level: when the mind isn't paying full attention to the sensation of food—its taste, scent, texture, and presentation—then eating itself becomes less satisfying. And a key way to compensate for getting less pleasure or gratification from food is to continue to eat more and more. The result? Mindless task snacking is likely to lead to eating more and enjoying it less.

In contrast, there's evidence that paying attention to food while you eat affects how your body metabolizes it in a positive, beneficial way. Because your mind is focused solely on eating, more digestive juices are recruited, starting with saliva. And because eating mindfully slows down the speed with which you eat, you're optimizing the digestive juices in your stomach; in fact, the entire digestive process is enhanced.

Metabolism of Mindfulness

Can the awareness with which you eat really make a difference to your health and well–being, to the way in which you metabolize your food? Or, vice versa, does eating while task snacking actually impair your ability to absorb food?

To find out whether eating mindfully is really beneficial to diges–tion, researcher Donald Morse, a physician and professor emeritus at Temple University in Philadelphia, designed a unique study to assess whether eating mindfully versus eating while distracted or stressed (task snacking) makes a difference to metabolism. He designed his experiment this way: one group of female college students would meditate for five minutes before eating cereal (a food high in car–bohydrates), while another group would distract themselves with mental arithmetic before eating the cereal (a form of task snacking). Afterward, when Dr. Morse and his team measured both groups' saliva (where metabolism of food begins), he discovered that those who meditated mindfully before eating produced 22 percent more of the digestive enzyme alpha–amylase.

There are two significant implications. Because alpha–amylase helps you digest and metabolize carbohydrates in carbohydrate–

dense foods (such as potatoes, bread, and cereal) as well as B vitamins (of which there are eight), if you eat while task snacking you're likely to absorb fewer nutrients than you need for your mind–body to function optimally. The study also "shows that there's a real benefit to having a leisurely meal," speculates Morse. "The decrease in alpha–amylase production is just the tip of the iceberg. When you gulp down your food, your entire digestive system is affected." Not only does task snacking have long–term implications for your digestion, but Morse's findings also imply that if you make subtle changes in the awareness you bring to food so that you're eating mindfully (doing one thing at a time—eating when you eat, working when you work), you're more likely to stop overeating and gaining weight.[3]

Medical Meditation

In Chapter 2, "Jettison Judgment," we introduced the concept of meditation as a way to transcend this overeating style. An integral aspect of – and Eastern healing systems (such as India's Ayurveda), meditation initially emerged in and penetrated Western science in the 1970s with the publication of physician Herbert Benson's pioneering and now–classic book *The Relaxation Response*. Director Emeritus of the Benson–Henry Institute for Mind Body Medicine (BHI) at Massachusetts General Hospital, Benson was the first person to doc–ument scientifically the deeply calming effects of meditation on the body's autonomic nervous system.

The innovative path he took to this realization is fascinating. Benson's journey began in India, where he went to do research with meditating monks in the Himalayan Mountains. As part of his experiment, he placed wet sheets on the monks, who then entered into deep meditation. The altitude was high and the weather was freezing. Under such circumstances, most of us would expect the water–drenched sheets to freeze and the monks themselves to be too uncomfortably cold to continue. But that isn't what happened. Instead, steam started to rise from the sheets covering the meditating monks, so much so that both the sheets and the monks actually dried off without freezing or getting cold.

What Benson and his team discovered was that with enough skill at meditation (for years, the monks had meditated for hours each day), human beings can control their body temperatures to an extraordinary degree. After returning to Harvard, Benson conducted more studies on the deeply calming effects of meditation. With the Harvard imprimatur, his studies led to the discovery that simple meditation techniques can profoundly calm the body's nervous system; ergo, Benson's "relaxation response" and the birth of mind–body medicine.[4]

Since Benson's findings about meditating monks in India, the field of meditation has evolved to include the practice of Medical Meditation. Proven effective by scientific studies, its unique focus is on concentration and how it can change your body, mind, and soul, in the process bringing you to a calm state of mind that can heal multidimensionally. And this includes turning to mindfulness meditation to overcome the tide of overeating and related weight gain. But before we tell you about groundbreaking research in the emerging field of mindfulness meditation as an antidote to task snacking and other eating disorders, we'd like to introduce you to a more in–depth understanding of what it means to eat mindfully. As you'll see, by focusing your awareness on food and eating, you're infusing yourself with a meditative sensibility that quiets the mind, soothes the soul . . . and begins to banish binge eating.

The "Tea Mind"

Following Benson's work, molecular biologist Jon Kabat–Zinn created a mindfulness meditation model and program used today in institutions ranging from Kabat–Zinn's Stress Reduction Clinic at the University of Massachusetts Medical School to hundreds of hospitals and clinics, corporations, sports teams, and prisons worldwide. A meditator himself since 1966, Kabat–Zinn developed his technique to give people an experiential, hands–on sense of what it means to meditate mindfully. Patients referred to his clinic for ailments ranging from stress to heart disease have reaped the rewards with a unique Buddhist–based meditation structured around the ordinary experience of eating. Kabat–Zinn calls it the "raisin meditation."

As Kabat–Zinn guides participants through his raisin meditation, they focus on all aspects of the experience of eating a single raisin: how it looks, smells, and feels; what happens in the mouth before, during, and after eating it; the motion and movement involved; the raisin's taste and texture; swallowing; and the role of breathing throughout the experience. From start to finish, it takes ten minutes to eat the raisin. And then the group is ready to begin the meditation process again with a second raisin.[5]

Later in this chapter, we'll guide you through this meditation (see "Raisin Consciousness"), but for now the key concept is the "consciousness" part of it: eating with moment–to–moment, non–judgmental attention to each element of the experience. What does it mean to have such focused attention on food? Is it simply paying attention to the ordinary experience of eating, or is it something more extraordinary? Or is it mundane? Ancient food wisdom offers some clues about what it means to be aware of being aware.

We vividly remember the moment we were introduced to the Chinese idea of "tea mind." It was during a visit to the Urasenke Foundation in San Francisco, where we'd been invited to observe students studying the Japanese Way of Tea (*chanoyu*). At any given time, we could hear the pouring of water, the clink of the lid on the iron kettle, or the whisking of the powdered green tea in water as it turned into a light, frothy brew. Surrounded by the timeless refine–ment of *chanoyu*, we realized that as much as it is an actual ceremony, it is also a consciousness, a "mentality of elegance," an experiential adventure that unfolds along with the passing moments.

Creating the alchemical brew with this kind of consciousness is a path to tea mind. With roots in Taoism, it means that—like tea—a person's mind is limitless, and a part of everything. As with the raisin meditation, accessing tea mind calls for drinking tea using all your senses, and more.[6] While Taoism provided the aesthetic ideals, it was a Zen Buddhist sect that integrated many Taoist doctrines into Japan's Way of Tea as it is practiced today. This appreciation of aesthetics is evident in the placement of flowers, the profound simplicity of the pottery, the architecture of the teahouse, and of course the tea powder itself. So integral is a refined consciousness to the Way of

Tea in Japanese culture that the concept has infiltrated the language through the word *chajin*, describing a person who has internalized the meditative awareness of tea mind. Observing the visible and invisible elements as they play together to satisfy the senses makes you less prone to overeat, in contrast to the busyness inherent in task snacking.

A Feel-Good Feedback Loop

Can the ephemeral, meditative sensibility inherent in the "unseeable principles" of tea mind and meditation make a difference to your weight and well-being? And if so, in what way? To answer these questions, researchers have begun to delve into the ancient discipline of mindfulness meditation to explore its potential to manage eating disorders. The idea has its roots in the growing field of brain research. In one of the first scientific studies done in the late 1960s on the meditating brain, psychiatrist Gregg Jacobs of Harvard Medical School recorded the EEGs (brain waves) of both meditators and another group of subjects who'd been given books on tape to listen to as a way to relax. Over the next few months, Jacobs noted that the meditators had lower activity in the parietal lobe section of the brain. When this sensory section of the brain shuts down, it's possible to feel fewer "boundaries" and in turn to feel more connected to, and one with, the universe.[7]

The meditating brain doesn't literally shut down; rather, it slows the receipt of information and keeps it from entering the part of the brain that orients us to time and space. More brain-imaging studies by Richard Davidson at the University of Wisconsin–Madison demonstrated that when you meditate regularly, the brain reorients from a right- prefrontal mindset of stress and discontent to a left-prefrontal disposition of relaxation and joy.[8] This is intriguing in terms of task snacking, because it explains how your brain produces the relaxation response Herbert Benson discovered among meditators; it is also another perspective about the profound way in which eating mindfully reduces stress and, in turn, diminishes overeating.

Meditation for Managing Binge Eating

What do mindfulness and meditation have to do with eating, task snacking, and your weight? A lot. In our research on the seven over−eating styles, the more our study participants reduced their task snacking, the more they reduced their weight—suggesting that you eat less when you focus on your food and the process of eating than when you are task snacking. The field of psychology is in its infancy in doing experiments that demonstrate the impact of mindfulness meditation and its link to weight loss, but there are some examples. Let us tell you about three of them.

In the 1980s Jean Kristeller of Indiana State University, where she is psychology professor emeritus and former director of the Center for the Study of Health, Religion, and Spirituality, began to use medita−tion to help patients de−stress with Benson's relaxation response. Then, inspired by Kabat−Zinn's raisin meditation, she turned her attention to meditation as a vehicle for helping people with compulsive eating problems. Over time she developed her Mindfulness−Based Eating Awareness Training (MB−EAT), a comprehensive nine−week pro−gram that integrates the experience of food and eating with "inner" and "outer" wisdom. The program is replete with meditative exercises that address hunger and satiety, forgiveness, and connecting to the inner wisdom that signals whether you're full and satisfied or hungry, with an appetite for a particular food. MB−EAT focuses on finding satisfaction in quality, not quantity.

To find out whether her MB−EAT program could help women with eating and weight problems, Kristeller recruited eighteen obese women, ages twenty−five to sixty−two. Each met the criteria of the American Psychiatric Association's *Diagnostic and Statistical Manual of Mental Disorders* (DSM−IV) for Binge Eating Disorder (BED), defined as recurrent episodes of out−of−control eating twice a week or more for six months or longer. The intervention focused on three forms of meditation: general mindfulness meditation, eating medita−tion, and mini−meditations.

With the general meditation, participants were taught to develop focused attention and awareness of an object, such as food. They would do this simply by noting their thoughts, emotions, or bodily sensations, then returning their attention to their breathing when they noticed their thoughts straying. This practice teaches individuals to observe the contents of the mind and the sensations of the body, without judgment, and at the same time to learn detached awareness. The eating meditation applied the general mindfulness meditation approach to more specific behaviors, beliefs, and emotions associated with food intake; again, emphasis was on retaining detached aware— ness. To do meditations, participants were instructed to take a few moments to stop and become aware of their thoughts and feelings prior to meals, or when the urge to binge surfaced.

After learning these techniques, participants met once a week for six weeks. For the first twenty minutes of each session, they dis— cussed their progress and any difficulties experienced during the prior week. Next they focused on a specific theme related to overcoming binge eating—becoming aware of binge triggers, hunger and satiety, self—forgiveness, relapse prevention, and exercises in eating mind— fully. Homework included daily meditation, either directed on tape or self—guided, and mindful—eating exercises.

At the end of the six weeks, Kristeller concluded that the program was, indeed, beneficial. Three weeks prior to starting the intervention, most women binged an average of five times each week. After three weeks of learning and practicing mindfulness meditation in prepa— ration for the study, the women lowered their average number of bingeing episodes to 3.9. And when the six—week program ended, the average number of binges was less than one (.9) per week.[9] Just as encouraging, when Kristeller did a three—week follow—up, she dis— covered the women were still benefiting, with bingeing episodes less than twice (1.6) weekly. In other words, bingeing behavior continued after the study, but there were far fewer episodes than when the study had started. Significantly, emotions that often sparked a bingeing episode, such as depression and anxiety, decreased. Kristeller's find— ings were so encouraging that the Center for Complementary and Alternative Medicine at the National Institutes of Health funded the psychologist and her team to do a similar nine—week program to examine how mindfulness meditation can promote weight loss.[10]

It may seem paradoxical that as the women in Kristeller's study let go of trying to control their eating, they gained more control over their binge eating in terms of doing it less often. A possible explanation is that when you do mindfulness meditation, you learn to detach yourself from the random impulse to binge and then act on it by eating. Mindfulness meditation empowers you to disconnect that circuit in the brain that attaches an emotion with a certain behavior sequence (bingeing). This suggests that if you have a negative feeling and want to binge, doing mindfulness meditation puts space between your feelings and bingeing; you realize that feelings come and go, and you don't necessarily have to act on them. You obtain a sense of control over bingeing and are empowered to turn to it as a coping mechanism less often.

Meditation and Your Weight
A first—of—its kind study that sheds light on the meditation/weight equation was conducted by researchers at Dr. Dean Ornish's Preventive Medicine Research Institute (PMRI) in Sausalito, California. The study, rooted in work Ornish did throughout the 1980s and 1990s, put meditation on the map by including it as part of a comprehensive program to reverse heart disease through lifestyle changes alone—stress management (meditation and yoga); a no—fat—added, plant—based diet; exercise; and group support—without drugs or surgery. Ornish's research was pioneering because it was substantive and sound and was published in prestigious medical journals, ranging from the *Journal of the American Medical Association* to *The Lancet* and other peer—reviewed journals.[11]

Following the publication of Ornish's reversal research, many health professionals contacted him wanting to know which components of the program contributed the most to reversing heart disease. Was it the low—fat diet? The stress—management techniques? Perhaps it was the exercise, or could it be the group support? Or was it the combination of all the components, working synergistically, that brought the benefits? Ornish and his research team decided to find out.

"Clearly, a study testing each component separately would offer much−needed information that could help many," medical psy−chologist Gerdi Weidner, PhD, told us. We talked with Weidner, vice president and director of research at PMRI, to learn about the results of the study firsthand. Formerly a professor of psychology and pre−ventive medicine at the State University of New York at Stony Brook, Weidner met co−author Larry in 1992 in Hannover, Germany, where he was presenting the Ornish reversal program at the International Society of Behavioral Medicine Conference. Larry was PMRI director of research for more than eighteen years prior to Weidner's taking over the position. At the time of the presentation, we were living in Germany, replicating Ornish's lifestyle research at a 350−bed cardiovascular clinic.

Continued Weidner, "With more than 850 patients with heart disease (both male and female) who have been enrolled in the Ornish program for at least three months, we now have a great opportu−nity to investigate the individual and joint contribution of life−style changes to coronary risk factors that are recommended by the Ornish program. In our new study, the Multi−Site Cardiac Lifestyle Intervention Program (MCLIP), we studied these patients in order to investigate the degree to which changing one's lifestyle behaviors (lowering dietary fat and increasing exercise and stress management practices of meditation and yoga) can improve risk factors linked with heart disease, such as weight, cholesterol levels, and depression and hostility."

Patients and their spouses met in groups twice weekly for three months, Weider said, for a total of 104 hours, to learn about the low−fat diet, exercise, and stress−management techniques including yoga sessions that ended with about ten minutes of meditation. During their time apart, participants were asked to practice stress manage−ment for one hour per day, with the option of doing this by listening to meditation tapes.[12]

Not surprisingly, results revealed that all three intervention modalities (diet, stress management, and exercise) played a posi−tive role in lowering risk factors for heart disease. For task snackers, though, what's most relevant are three key findings. The first revealed that *the amount of time each person spent meditating was directly linked with the amount of weight lost, regardless of whether participants changed their dietary fat intake or their exercise habits.* In fact, those who did *not* change their dietary fat intake but increased their stress management practice by as much as six hours per week lost an average of almost twenty pounds for men and more than twelve pounds for women.

Second and equally pertinent, the greatest weight loss was achieved by those who increased their yoga and meditation while they *decreased* their intake of dietary fat. Specifically, those who increased their stress manage−ment practice to six hours per week *and* reduced their dietary fat intake to 15 percent calories from fat lost an average of about twenty−seven pounds for men and twenty pounds for women at the end of three months.

The third key finding goes against the conventional energy−in (food), energy−out (exercise) guidelines: in the Multi−Site Cardiac Lifestyle Intervention Program, an increase in exercise didn't con−tribute any further to the amount of weight loss. Rather, it was the amount of time participants meditated and the degree to which they lowered their dietary fat intake that brought the best results.

Although the exact reasons stress management leads to weight loss are unclear, Weidner offers some possible explanations about why meditation may contribute to weight loss. Meditation directs your awareness away from external cues (such as eating lunch at noon, when you "should") to focusing your attention internally (eating when you're actually feeling hungry). It may also diminish stress−related eating (discussed in detail in the next chapter)—turning to food when you're feeling anxious or upset.

As Ornish says: practicing all components of his program is the key to achieving beneficial health outcomes—including weight loss. Adds Weidner, "In our analyses, increases in stress management and medita−tion contributed not only to weight loss but also to reductions in diabetic risk and hostile feelings [a risk factor for heart disease]. And less dietary fat intake added further to weight loss and to reductions in perceived stress. Add exercise to the equation, and your ability to burn energy (calories) increases."[13] So, too, with *Make Weight Loss Last*: optimize and implement all the antidotes to the overeating styles discussed in this book, including mindful eating, and you're more likely to lose more weight.

Raisin Consciousness

The practice of mindful awareness is rooted in one of Buddhism's earliest sutras, or teachings. Called the Mindfulness Sutra, it describes how to cultivate judgment—free, impartial awareness of what you are doing during each moment. The raisin meditation that Jon Kabat—Zinn teaches his patients is based on Buddhist wisdom he learned from Jack Kornfield, one the West's leading Buddhist teachers. Here's a version you can experience for yourself. To get the most benefit, first read through the steps before doing the exercise.

1. Sit in a comfortable chair and set a small bowl filled with rai—sins on a table next to you.

2. Select one raisin from the bowl.

3. Look at the raisin as if it were an alien object you had never seen before. As you look at it, imagine it in its original form as a grape, growing in the sunshine surrounded by air, earth, and water.

4. Continuing to look at the raisin, describe what you see: its texture, color, shape, and anything else that comes to mind.

5. Bring the raisin up to your nose. Smell it. Describe its scent.

6. As you smell the raisin, are you experiencing any changes in your mouth, in your saliva, as you anticipate eating the raisin?

7. How does the raisin feel? Describe it.

8. Become aware of your body and the hand that is holding the raisin. Consider how your hand knows how to hold the raisin, how to bring it up toward your nose.

9. Bring the raisin toward your lips, then place it in your mouth. What motion is your tongue doing? Your jaw? Your teeth? Your cheek?

10. Now focus all your attention in your mouth. Bite into the raisin slowly . . .and begin to chew . . . slowly. Stop after three chews. On which side of your mouth are you chewing? What are your tongue, jaw, teeth, and cheek doing now?

11. Describe the taste you're experiencing.

12. Continue to chew, but don't swallow the raisin. Do you notice a difference in the taste? What is the texture like?

13. Are you tempted to swallow yet? Observe what's happening in your mouth as you prepare to swallow. Now swallow the raisin. Imagine it in your stomach, and acknowledge that your body is one raisin heavier.

14. Can you "taste" your breath now? Focus your attention on your breath as you inhale and exhale slowly.

15. Remain focused on your breath as you continue to inhale and exhale. Now, simply become silent. If you notice your mind wandering, bring your attention back to your breath. For the next five, ten, fifteen minutes, or longer, continue to focus on your breathing.

Congratulations! You've just experienced mindfulness meditation. For the greatest benefit, meditating twenty to thirty minutes each day is optimal. If setting aside special time to meditate is challenging for you, consider turning each meal or snack into an opportunity to eat mindfully. In Chapter 12, "Winning Weight–Loss Strategies," we'll show you how to overcome obstacles so you can do so each time you eat. But for now, take a cue from time–tested food wisdom: pay attention to every food–related act, every sensation and perception, for its own sake—to stay in the moment. From planning and preparing a meal to serving, eating, and clean–up, take your actions off auto–pilot and, instead, commit to being fully aware of what your hands, mouth, and mind are experiencing moment to moment— for in the witnessing lies the antidote to task snacking.

Other Simple Strategies

Cultivating mindfulness—paying attention intentionally—empowers you to slow down long enough to experience the subtleties of food. This is beneficial, because when you focus on your food, you're not task snacking; you're simply tasting your food and savoring the experience of eating. In Chapter 8, "Feed the Senses," we'll tell you more about the philosophy of the "six tastes" espoused by Eastern healing systems. Right now, though, you can reap rewards by focusing on the flavors in food each time you eat.

Savor flavor. The next time you eat a mixed meal, such as a salad or stew made with varied ingredients, bring your attention to your mouth; then, as you chew, try to identify the flavors in your food. Is it mostly sweet, or is salt the major flavor? Did you experience a burst of flavor at the first bite? Are you still enjoying the taste of the food after the second and third bites?

Take tea time. Another way to approach your journey of mindfulness is to perceive of tea as an opportunity to balance the five elements of metal (minerals in the soil that help create tea leaves); wood (the tea plant); water (that brings tea back to life); fire (the sun that heats the water); and earth (the mother of tea and material for teapots). Followers of Japan's Way of Tea (often called the Japanese Tea Ceremony) believe that when the elements are balanced and in harmony, they create a form of perfection. The next time you savor a cup of tea, think about whether you can see and taste each element with each sip. Consider bringing a similar consciousness to all the beverages you consume during the day.

Move into mindfulness. There are three distinct steps to take to replace task snacking with conscious, intentional awareness:

1. *Intentionality*: don't just think about doing it; make a decisive choice to focus on the food before you when you're eating.

2. *Commitment*: act on your intention. Carry it out by gently letting go of feelings, thoughts, and activities that may be interfering with your intention and commitment to mindfulness.

3. *Focus*: with intention and commitment to mindfulness, keep your attention on the food or food–related activities you are experiencing.

Focus on Food

Taking the time to "eat when you eat," and in this way to truly taste and savor food, is the key to overcoming task snacking and avoiding weight gain. Here's the antidote to task snacking:

Task Snacking Rx: Bring moment-to-moment nonjudgmental awareness to each aspect of the meal.

Replace eating while doing other things—shopping, working, or watching television—with moment–to–moment nonjudgmental awareness of each aspect of your meal, and you're on the path to making weight loss last.

Chapter 4

Access Your Appetite

In the twenty–five–plus years that Barbara Birsinger has been studying emotional eating, she has come to believe that emotional eaters seek food in an attempt to manage unpleasant feelings such as depression, anxiety, or anger. When negative emotions emerge, emotional eaters turn to food as a distraction, as a way to run away from, and to numb, these feelings. They aren't eating because they are hungry; they are eating in response to disagreeable emotions.

Birsinger knows a lot about emotional eating—both person–ally and as a professional who is a registered dietitian (RD) with a doctorate in theology, spiritual healing, and energy medicine. Her epiphany came from her own early struggles with emotional eating, which developed into an eating disorder that she successfully over–came. Her insights emerged a few years after she graduated from the University of California, Berkeley, where she obtained a mas–ter's degree in public health nutrition. Emotional eating—and over–coming it—meant so much to her that it was the focus of the research she did for her dissertation.

How did Birsinger win her battle with emotional eating? When we talked with her, she explained that she didn't want to live her life focused on food and feelings. She wanted a balanced life that included marriage and children—both of which have now been a part of her life for many years. Clearly her profound compassion for the millions who struggle with food and weight, and her deep interest in nutrition and optimal eating, have a lot to do with her own personal success.

During our discussion, Birsinger talked about her personal experience with her own food− and weight−related struggles; she also revealed a lot about her research on overcoming emotional eating and overeating. We wanted to speak with Birsinger, specifically, because we share a strong conviction that optimal eating and normal weight aren't achieved via a list of "do and don't" instructions; they are the side effects that come naturally when you perceive food and eating as a path that leads to physical, emotional, spiritual, and social well−being. In other words, your relationship with eating is transformed from a problem into a solution when you allow food to heal you in every way.

We talked for a little over six hours. The following excerpt of that conversation is just a fraction of the story Birsinger shared with such concern and care. Her insights provide a clear portrait of how she transformed a life of emotional eating and yo−yo weight problems into one based on a solid foundation of mind−body balance.

There was a lot of love in my family, and thankfully I always knew that. But along with an abundance of love, there was an abun−dance of food. I grew up on a farm in the Midwest. My father was a veterinarian, and my mother, a housewife in the 1950s, gar−dened, cooked, baked, and canned. Food was plentiful and always available, and there were few rules around it. We ate three meals a day of delicious, fresh, homemade food, which included our own meats and dairy, and fresh fruits and vegetables. We could snack freely on freshly baked bread, fruit pies, and cookies, all of which were stocked in a huge pantry to which I had easy access.

My father died of a long illness when I was a child, and his death was a taboo topic. Growing up in a family that didn't acknowledge feelings, I experienced considerable emotional stress. We moved from the farm at the time I started middle school, and this is when I started to develop a problem with food and body image. In junior high school, I was teased about being too skinny; after all, people were judging how I looked all the time. My girl−friend and I decided to eat double lunches to gain weight, but we just got taller, not more curvy.

We moved again, this time to an affluent community, just when I started high school, and it was lonely. I didn't know any—body and felt that I didn't fit in. I gained twenty—five pounds in the first year. About this time, I met a girl who was dieting, so I decided to try it, too. I rode my bike seven miles to school each day, surviving on lettuce—and yes, I lost weight. It amazed me that no one noticed or was aware of the danger I was putting myself in with constant dieting and fasting. At the same time, I studied hard and I liked school, but I hated the social and competitive aspects of high school, so I graduated in three years instead of four. This meant that I started UC, Berkeley, at sixteen, and being younger than the other students and emotionally unprepared, college was stressful. I wasn't prepared emotionally; as with high school, it was lonely and isolating.

By the time I was eighteen, I had been dieting for several years. Now I started to get gastric reflux symptoms: food wouldn't digest and it would start to come up through my esophagus. After many doctor visits, and not being able to stop the reflux, I began to use it as a weight—control method, and later I started to binge eat. My bingeing was related to the emotional issues I was going through. It was hard for me to stomach the stress of being so young at a huge university. Having inadequate emotional support at school and at home, I was stuffing down my feelings; after all, I was taught to keep them in with the hope that they would go away; there just weren't any other acceptable choices in my family.

When I started thinking about how to stop binge eating, I realized that when I felt upset or anxious, food helped to calm me down and make me feel better. When I was overwhelmed by my emotions it felt like a tidal wave, and I would binge to cope. The foods I binged on were foods that had been abundant in our home while I was growing up: scrumptious cinnamon twists, homemade bread with butter and jam, chocolate chip cookies, and apple and peach pies.

Then, when I was about twenty—six, I sat down in silence one day out of deep despair with my situation. I knew I wanted to stop. I wanted a different life. I didn't want to feel like an imposter with a secret life anymore. This was in the 70s, and I had gone to therapists, but at the time they didn't yet know about emotional eating or eating disorders, and the doctors I saw couldn't help, either. I realized that, inevitably, it was up to me and me alone to help myself.

When I looked at the pattern of everything that contributed to my bingeing, clearly the emotional component was the strongest reason. Binges were in response to emotions and feelings I wasn't capable of dealing with in the moment, and bingeing was how I would get relief. I had spent ten years running from feelings I now realized I could actually live through without bingeing. Another turning point was identifying the amount of food I could eat without having a reflux response. I decided to start eating without bingeing, which included stocking my shelves with all of the foods I grew up with—many of which had become illegal by dieting standards or were unhealthy according to nutrition textbooks. It was liberating to know that I didn't have to eat all the food at once, because I could trust my body with the amount it wanted—and I could have it again, anytime. I might have more of whatever it was I wanted within an hour or two after eating, but most often I didn't want more.

In retrospect, I realize I was relearning what we now call Intuitive Eating. I was learning to tune in to internal cues to guide me to knowing whether I was eating because I was hungry, or if I had an appetite for a particular food, or if I was satiated and no longer really wanted to eat. We're all born with the ability to eat this way, to look within to know what our minds and bodies need and want, and how much to eat; to be with ourselves and our feelings and not stuff them down with food. I also stopped exercising compulsively to keep my weight down if I overate. I wanted to be healthy and to have an active life with children and grandchildren—not to get rid of calories. I wanted to end the eating disorders way more than I was concerned about being fat. It was then that I began a working on emotional and spiritual issues.[1]

Why was Birsinger able to take a sudden intuitive leap of under—standing and transform a ten—year habit of emotional eating into normal, optimal eating? How, exactly, did she create such profound, meaningful change in her relationship to food, eating, and weight—changes that stayed with her for life? And if Birsinger can do it, can the millions of us who struggle with the same issues have the same success? Birsinger's transformation gives us clues about how to change, while her research on the topic, discussed later in the chapter, provides empirical evidence that decoding your emotions is the key to success. But first, let's visit the world of emotional eaters, those who have suc—cessfully left it, and the science that has supported their journey.

Feeding Negative Feelings with Food

For Ann, nighttime binge eating starts after work with a trip to the supermarket to buy bags of corn chips and chunks of her favorite chocolate. Then she heads home, changes into comfortable clothes, and turns on the TV. Settling into bed surrounded by her favorite foods, she begins what she describes as "zoning out"—eating until she feels calmer—often to the point of falling in and out of sleep well before bedtime. Although this is a typical evening for Ann, three hours after starting her binge, she is amazed to find that she has fin—ished all the food. On a not—quite—conscious level, she senses the chips and chocolate allay her anxiety in some way. She's also con—cerned about these binges because she wants to lose fifty pounds and stop zoning out, but she hasn't figured out how to accomplish this. Dieting hasn't helped, nor have willpower or the techniques she's read about in self—help books. In the meantime, Ann remains vaguely depressed and distressed, and dependent on food binges to manage her darker moods.

Theories have abounded for decades about the causes of all kinds of chemical and behavioral addictions, from hard—core drugs to food. (See the Introduction for more about food addiction.) Cassandra Vieten, PhD, is a clinical psychologist and researcher who special—izes in mind—body medicine and behavioral disorders at California Pacific Medical Center Research Institute in San Francisco and at the Institute of Noetic Sciences in nearby Petaluma. She believes "negative affect" may be the unifying factor in overeating, disordered eating, and an addiction to food influenced by genetics, environment, brain chemistry, and family dynamics.

"Negative affect is distress that can be conscious or unconscious, physiological, emotional, psychological, and/or spiritual," Vieten told us. "Distress is part of life, but some experience greater amounts of it, or are more highly sensitive to it due to their hardwiring or upbringing. Others experience stress as intolerable because they haven't developed the capacity to endure negative feelings." Indeed, our research showed that negative emotions—especially depression, boredom, and frustration—are what drive impulse eating and cravings; they are the strongest predictor of overeating and ensuing weight gain.

Bad, worrisome, anxious, unpleasant feelings are clearly a key aspect of negative affect for many, but for others—like Ann, who fixates on food for less conscious reasons—suppressed, unexpressed, or unidentified feelings can be part of the negative affect picture that manifests itself in emotional eating. "Some people can't or won't express themselves even when they know they are experiencing fear or anger. Still others often feel nondescript distress, but they can't say why, nor can they put a name on it," said Vieten.

When a person experiences undifferentiated negative affect, it may convey itself through bodily sensations, such as a tight stomach or muscular tension. If ongoing or extreme, these physical feelings can translate into a sense that you're not going to survive the emotions. Unfortunately, many treat (self-medicate) these sensations by over-eating certain foods that actually can alter their mental state. Because overeating can halt the distress—for the moment—it can become a powerful reinforcer. But it's possible to build up a tolerance, and to need more and more food to feel good again. When this happens, you're not really eating to feel better; you may be bingeing just to feel normal. The good news is that there are also ways to build your tolerance to distress—ways to relate to it, contain it, and cope with it—so that you are less and less driven to engage in self-medicating behaviors.[2]

Of Food and Mood

Although the term "emotional eating" wasn't in the culture in 1960 when Overeaters Anonymous (OA) was founded, "HALT" was already in use by Alcoholics Anonymous and was borrowed by OA. An organization that offers a twelve–step recovery program for compulsive overeating and other eating disorders, OA warned its members against becoming too Hungry, too Angry, too Lonely, or too Tired— because when you're feeling HALT emotions and you're an overeater, such emotions may trigger a binge.

Feeling HALT emotions means you are more likely to seek *false* relief by abusing yourself with food: become too hungry, and too many cookies may override healthful food choices, chomping on chips may suppress anger, ice cream may soothe loneliness, or you may befriend French fries when you feel tired. Whatever the emo– tional upset, in place of giving (gifting?) yourself what you really need, you choose food and compulsive overeating as your solution.

OA was way ahead of its time—and science—when it linked HALT emotions with the tendency of overeaters to turn to food for comfort. Today, health professionals often use the term "self–medi– cate" to describe the drive behind eating to cope and to feel better when unpleasant emotions such as depression and anxiety emerge.

The idea that the food you eat can actually medicate your mood and vice versa—that your mood may motivate you to make certain food choices—was given the scientific stamp of approval in the 1970s when Judith Wurtman, PhD, a scientist at the Massachusetts Institute of Technology, uncovered a fascinating facet of the emotional eating enigma. Call it nutritional neuroscience, psychoneuroimmunology, the study of food and mood, or psychological nutrition (our term for it), Wurtman launched a new field of nutrition research that has confirmed what OA and many of us know intuitively: *what* you eat affects your mind and mood, your tendency to pile on pounds, even the quality of your life.

When Wurtman and her husband, Richard Wurtman, MD, also at MIT, first linked food with mood, it was based on their discovery that both naturally occurring sugar and starch in carbohydrate foods (such as potatoes and whole grains) and sugar added to food products (such as cookies and cake) elevate a powerful chemical in your brain called serotonin. Even more fascinating was their discovery about the impact serotonin and other neurotransmitters (substances that pass information from cell to cell in the brain) have on your every mood, emotion, and food craving.

For instance, about twenty minutes after you eat a carbohydrate–rich food, your brain releases serotonin; in turn, you feel more relaxed and calm. Want to feel more perky? Consume a lean, high–protein food such as fish, and the substance that's released (norepinephrine) lets you feel more awake and energetic (unlike the kick you get from caffeine, you're not stimulated, just more alert).[3]

Here is where the food–mood link really gets interesting. Since the Wurtmans' research, we've had strong clinical evidence that carbohydrates can be calming, protein–based foods can perk you up, and certain fats in food end up as endorphins—substances in the brain that produce pleasurable feelings. But now we also know that the sugary and sweet or crunchy and fried *processed food products* that emotional eaters most often choose to get a serotonin high actually contribute to *deficiencies* in certain vitamins and minerals that can cause your emotions to plummet, leading to a serious case of the doldrums.

In this way, the food–mood syndrome becomes a vicious emotional cycle. You're feeling down, so you reach for, say, a prepackaged brownie. Sure, the brownie's sugar and white flour carb content will soothe and calm you, but its high sugar content has a hidden side effect: it actually depletes some nutrients that could help combat depression. The sweet concoction may somehow soothe your soul, but isn't it ironic that at the same time, it may also contribute to anxiety, depression, and other unpleasant emotions? To bust the blues with food, look over the "B Wise" tips toward the end of this chapter.

Tapping into Transformation

While most of us try to cope with our emotions, food, and weight with the food–fretting eating style—dieting, counting calories or carbs, measuring portion size, restricting or avoiding foods, and continuing to worry about our weight—those who transition successfully, permanently, and effectively from emotional eating to optimal eating and weight, as Barbara Birsinger did, reject food fretting. Instead, they tap into their emotions, identify their real needs, and then act on what will satisfy those needs. Often what brings true satisfaction has nothing to do with food, although sometimes it does.

There is an excellent example of the life−transforming dynamics that allowed Birsinger to stop food fretting and bingeing, and transi−tion from being an emotional eater to an optimal eater, in the work of Eckhart Tolle, author of *The Power of Now.* Prior to his complete change, he lived as a hermit, immersed in a depressed and anxiety−filled frame of mind; his emotional pain was so all−invasive that he considered ending his life. And then, at the depth of his despair, he realized that his miserable self and the "I," the "owner" of his miser−able self, weren't two different people; that only the "I" was real.

Fully conscious and stunned at this realization, he felt "intense fear," so much so that he began to shake. At the same time, he was guided to "resist nothing," and instead to become one with simply being alive. And then he fell into a deep sleep. The next morning, Tolle awakened filled with a deep understanding and appreciation of life itself, and the wonder of his existence. Something profoundly transcendent had happened to him.

Immersed in his bliss, Tolle spent two years living on park benches, simply being "in a state of the most intense joy." During this time he realized that regardless of ever−changing circumstances, situations, or emotions—positive or negative, happy or sad, good or bad, painful or joyful—he lived with an underlying sense of peace, calmness, and connection to a larger whole; that the "mystery of life," if you will, is constant. And this realization is what gave him—and continues to give him—deep peace of mind.[4]

It sounds so simple, doesn't it? Just access the truth that's within you to transform emotions that lead to overeating into a blissful, peaceful life without weight worries. As you know and I know, for most of us making a shift in our way of being and seeing the world is neither instantaneous nor easy. Rather, changing from being *in the world* and feeding emotions with food to being *of the world* and feeling a connection to food and eating—or to any other joy−filled, intentionally chosen activity—is often a messy process that starts with small steps and lots of contemplation before we're able to take action.

What made Barbara Birsinger able to transform and grow from being an emotional eater into being a normal eater? Whether suddenly, or slowly over time, she was able to let go of and move beyond a limited sense of self and expand the vision of her purpose, destiny, and role in the universe. What especially sets her apart is that instead of accepting her eating disorder as it was, she was transformed when she felt passionate about moving beyond what she was *doing*, and instead somehow knew that she needed to *be* part of something bigger than herself. For Birsinger, this larger connection meant healing so that she could become a wife and mother, and this called for learning to *be* outside herself, to be other–oriented. By integrating and connecting her emotions, thoughts, dreams, and visions with the outside world, she ignited a spark that enabled her to launch the transformation to a more fulfilling, balanced, meaningful life.

Vieten offers this insight into transformation as a means of ending emotional eating: "Connecting to something deeper than your individual craving or desire can also be incredibly helpful. Not only can it empower you to ride the waves of craving, emotional and spiritual awareness can enable you to use intention and choice to decide how you want to live in the world."[5]

The Evolution of Emotional Eating

The specialty of emotional eating has come a long way since the 1960s when Overeaters Anonymous advised its members to HALT negative feelings of Hunger, Anger, Loneliness, and Tiredness.[6] Since then, a comprehensive emotional eating industry has evolved, replete with sound research, support groups, therapy options, and books. Barbara Birsinger didn't have these resources when she was a teenager and college student in the 1970s, struggling alone with her eating disorders. But, she recalls, some early clues were beginning to emerge about emotional eating and other eating disorders, clues indicating that eating disorders were coming out of the closet and into the culture.

Chocolate: Elixir of Love

No discussion about emotional eating, food and mood, and weight would be complete without pausing to savor the emotional ambrosia associated with choice chocolate. For centuries, chocolate has been lauded in literature, has been christened "food of the gods" with its botanical name (*Theobroma cacao*), and has flourished as a reputed aphrodisiac. The mystique of chocolate continues to be manifest in movies such as *Charlie and the Chocolate Factory*, *Like Water for Chocolate*, the 2001 Academy Award nominee *Chocolat*, and *Forrest Gump*, with its famous line, "Life is like a box of chocolates, you never know what you're gonna get." But as science continues to focus its microscope on chocolate, the more we *do* know what we're gonna get: emotional gratification and physical nourishment.

Today, science is verifying that chocolate offers more than alleged aphrodisiac powers and that it does, indeed, nourish both mind and body. The sugar, fat, and caffeine content of today's chocolate confections, combined with some of the naturally occurring chemicals in the cacao bean, has the power to enhance emotions and, perhaps, even heal the heart.

Consider what happens when you consume the sweet-and-creamy concoction of cocoa combined with sugar and fat: blues-busting endorphins, naturally occurring substances (hormones) in the brain that function as painkillers and produce pleasurable feelings, are released. Such mood enhancers are compounded by the *phenylethylamine* (PEA) in chocolate, a substance that likely enhances the release of endorphins. Indeed, the PEA released when you eat chocolate is the same PEA that produces its euphoric side effects when you fall in love. Add druglike components in chocolate such as caffeine and phenylethylamine, and you may have a recipe for "chocoholism."

Equally interesting is recent research about good-quality dark chocolate (which contains a high percentage of cocoa) presented to the European Society of Cardiology in Munich. Apparently dark chocolate's high levels of flavonoids—antioxidants that mop up artery-clogging chemicals in the body—may help reduce heart disease by improving the function of the endothelial cells in the arteries.

To get these benefits, choose up to two ounces of dark chocolate with a high cocoa content (70 percent or higher) each day.

In 1977, while doing their dietetic internship rotation at a local hospital, Birsinger and other students were told by the chief dietitian that she'd started to see patients—mostly girls—who wouldn't eat (signs of anorexia nervosa) or, if they did eat, would then throw up the food (the bingeing and purging syndrome of bulimia nervosa). "It was the first time I ever heard that others had my problem," Birsinger told me. "But what the chief dietitian was describing did more harm than good. Talking about the psychological profile of people with eating disorders, she described them as emotional cripples, as people who have huge issues with their overcontrolling mothers, and as people with low morals who lie and steal and can't be trusted. I remember feeling frozen and thinking that I could never ever tell anybody about this. Although I now know there is a diagnosis for what I was experiencing, neither health professionals nor I knew what it was at the time. I decided that I could not get help from my professional or medical community because they may have this misperception and misunderstanding about me and my eating problem. Not identifying with what my teacher was saying, and feeling that nobody would understand, I went underground and decided that I had to manage my eating issues myself. But they only got worse."

That is, until she put a permanent brake on them ten years later. "I was extremely lucky I was able to do this," Birsinger explains. "Because there is so much support and professional help today that would have eased much of my loneliness and pain, I wouldn't recommend that anyone struggling with eating issues try to solve them on their own. If help for my eating disorder had been available, it would have sped my recovery."[7]

Since then, Birsinger has turned her recovery program into a teaching tool that has helped many others. Birsinger was so convinced her method could help the millions of us who medicate our emotions with food that she did her doctoral dissertation on her method.[8] And her personal experience of recovery through intuitive eating—knowing without conscious reasoning when to eat, what to eat, and how much to eat, and what's optimal for an individual at any given time—would serve as a model for her research.

Birsinger's Decoding Emotional Eating

What's fascinating about emotional eating, of course, is that not all women and men succumb to feeding their emotions with food. Those who don't use food tend to replace the urge to splurge with dealing directly with their emotions. This idea of meeting emotional needs head on, instead of indirectly and symbolically through food, is exactly what intrigued Birsinger. Putting this insight into action had worked effectively for her, empowering her to end her emotional eating disorder.

Those who have looked into the causes of overeating and the reasons most of us fail at dieting agree that emotional factors play a large role. Emotional eating is such a powerful internal demon that it overrides our knowledge about what to eat and tyrannizes us in our weight loss plans. Aware of this when she began her study, Birsinger set out to do more than measure emotional eating: she was determined to develop a way to give people the skills they need to transform, and take control of, their emotional eating urges. Her core belief was that if emotional as well as physical, spiritual, and social needs could be filled directly, participants would be less likely to turn to food to cope, and managing eating and weight more effectively would be a side effect of her intervention.

There were several key considerations. Without following a prescribed diet, can adults self-regulate their eating by using intuitive tools? Can they learn to rely on their internal resources to improve their eating habits? Can they get the appropriate amount of calories and nutrients in their food, relying on their own internal resources and mind-body to eat optimally? It was time to find out.

To tease out the answers to her questions, Birsinger took a refreshingly novel approach, a comprehensive one that considered the full spectrum of emotional, spiritual, and social factors contributing to overeating. She all but ignored the more typical mono-focus on *what* to eat and its straitjacket of traditional dietary recommendations. Instead, she evaluated the effectiveness of an integrative healing approach to resolve disordered eating and weight issues. She randomly assigned 102 adult women, ages nineteen to seventy—six (median age: fifty—one), to either an intervention group or a control (waitlist) group. Fifty—four healthy adult women, interested in an alternative approach to eating and weight management, were in the intuitive eating group. Forty—eight participants in the delayed treatment group would eat what was normal for them during the study, then be trained in the intuitive eating method afterward.

Each group filled out questionnaires when the study started; after the eight—week program, they filled out the same questionnaires again so that changes, if any, could be measured. The questionnaires not only measured eating behaviors but also looked at the subtler emotional, spiritual, and social reasons why people overeat. Birsinger analyzed the varieties of internal and external factors prompting us to eat: intrinsic eating (eating in response to being bored, upset, anxious, depressed, or frustrated), extrinsic eating (eating in response to food that tastes good, or when you smell something delicious), and restrained eating (intentionally consuming fewer calories than your body needs). She measured restrained eating by asking respondents whether their eating was restrained when their weight was up. Another of the nuances Birsinger explored was the feelings that certain foods represented to each participant.

And then the program began. During this time, the intervention group received sixteen hours of experiential instruction and training designed by Birsinger. Topics included intuitive eating techniques (learning to identify the difference between physical hunger and symbolic hunger, the desire to eat without physical hunger); decoding of symbolic food cravings; mindfulness and nonjudgmental eating; abundance, consciousness, and environmental planning for optimal foods; practicing presence; joy of movement; self— and body—acceptance; and the influence of feminine and masculine archetypal energies on food and body issues.

Birsinger used a rich repository of teaching tools that included lectures and presentations; group, dyad, and triad discussions; question—and—answer sessions; guided imagery; journal exercises; right—

brain writing and drawing; expressive art and somatic movement activities; psycho−drama/role play; meditation and contemplative practice; myths, metaphors, storytelling; and the Inner Counselor and Symbolic Visualization Process. Her teaching methods were as diverse as the program she created, and the intervention was inten− sively interactive.

Was the effort worth it? Did participants obtain the benefits both Birsinger and they were hoping for? The results were in large part what Birsinger hoped to achieve. After learning Birsinger's techniques, participants were able both to maintain their weight and to prevent gaining it back. Those who lost the most weight had made the most changes in emotional eating, which suggests that overcoming this eating behavior is key.

The findings, though, reached far beyond weight, because those who received Birsinger's intensive, extensive, and comprehensive training in intuitive and integrative practices decreased their symbolic food cravings (eating for reasons other than hunger) and overeating behaviors. And there were other beneficial outcomes: fewer com− pulsive eating and dieting behaviors, less anxiety about eating, and a stronger sense of connection. Attitudes toward eating improved, as did acceptance of body image, self−esteem, spiritual well−being, and self− care practices (physical activity and emotional support, for example).[9]

Such encouraging results suggest that ongoing weight−loss suc− cess hinges on changing the whole matrix of physical, emotional, spiritual, and social factors involved in overeating. In the Introduction to this book we discussed the four facets of food (eating for physical, emotional, spiritual, and social well−being) and our Whole Person Nutrition Model and Program, the essence of which is overcoming the seven overeating styles, as the keys to achieving and maintaining optimal weight and well−being. Birsinger's findings support our eating−style research and its link to multidimensional well−being.

More studies need to be done to see whether those who partici− pated in Birsinger's program can maintain their improved relationship to food. The more important take−away message, though, is that a whole person nutrition approach—one that targets the multidimensional dis− ruptive emotions that drive us to overeat—seems to be more useful than focusing on just one eating style (such as food fretting) when it comes to providing a possible solution to America's obesity epidemic.

Transformation Strategies

Right now, you're at a turning point. You can decide to take care of your physical and symbolic hunger needs in an appropriate way. Or you can continue to turn to food to do the job. By choosing the path of transformation, you're deciding to feed your body, mind, and soul what they really need; in other words, you're giving yourself true nourishment. The following exercises may not resolve all your eating problems overnight, but they can be a helpful if you practice them each time the urge to splurge surfaces. The secret? Birsinger's "decoding process" shows you how to shed light on unmet intrinsic needs that may be at the root of disordered eating. And then, symbolically, she'll show you how to transform your craving by filling your needs with something other than food.

Birsinger has a strong conviction that there's a reason and a purpose for overeating. You're trying to take care of yourself on some level, to fill a need that's not getting cared for in another way. Food is available. It can do the job well, but it's only temporary—and there are side effects and consequences. If no effective self–care mechanisms are in place, your emotional eating isn't going to go away. The antidote? Develop the capacity to tolerate a range of unpleasant emotions. Birsinger offers the following two strategies for dealing with emotional eating: one for *physical* hunger, one for *symbolic* hunger.

Is Your Hunger Physical or Symbolic?

Overcoming overeating starts with discerning physical hunger from symbolic hunger. When you think of eating, is your desire to eat coming from physical hunger (located in your stomach) or symbolic hunger (eating for reasons other than physical nourishment)? Physical hunger is often experienced in the stomach, while symbolic hunger often manifests itself in the chest, throat, or mouth. In other words, *where* you're feeling hunger is a clue about whether the feeling is physical or symbolic.

Physical hunger. *How hungry are you?* Imagine the following sce-nario. You're at your desk and begin to think about eating. Ask yourself whether you're physically hungry in your body, or whether you have symbolic hunger. You realize you're actually hungry. Sitting at your desk and thinking of food is your cue to check in with your hunger level. On a scale of 1 to 10, identify your hunger level (1 is famished, 5 is neutral, and at 10 you are way overfed). You identify that you're at level 3, which means you've identifed that you're physically hungry and need to eat.

Decide what to eat and how much. Now decide what you want to eat. How much of it do you want? To know what your mind—body wants to eat, develop a mind—body connection. You can do this by checking in with your body before eating. To begin, ask your body what it wants. Doing this, Birsinger says, means eating from the neck *down* instead of the neck *up* (all in your mind)—where most people make decisions about what to eat.

Do the guided imagery visualization. Birsinger developed the guided imagery visualization exercise on the next page to provide the skills you need to make the mind—body connection, which in turn can empower you to dramatically change what and how you eat, forever. Practice it every time you eat.

Symbolic hunger. Now imagine this scenario. You're at your desk and you begin to think about eating. Ask yourself whether you're physically hungry in your body, or whether you have symbolic hunger. Okay, you're feeling anxious, you realize. No, you're not actually hungry. Your hunger is symbolic, not literal and physical. You really want chocolate chip cookies to help you cope with uncomfortable emotions. Even though you're not hungry, you're still wanting to eat. What's going on? You can't wait until you're hungry. If you can wait, great. Many can't, though, because emotional eating is an ingrained habit. If so . . . Birsinger suggests that you go to Step 2 of the Guided Imagery Visualization Exercise (see the sidebar).

If you could have anything you wanted, what would it be? The intensity of the emotion will determine whether you can wait or not. If nothing else will help, you may need to eat that cookie. Keep in mind, though, that by doing this process before you eat, you're becoming conscious of your needs and eating behaviors—without judgment. And such nonjudgmental awareness is a key step toward diminished overeating.

Guided Imagery Visualization Exercise

1. Inhale deeply, pause for two seconds, and exhale deeply, bringing your awareness from your head to your body. Notice air moving through your lungs. Notice the movement of your stomach expanding and contracting.

2. Imagine that you could have anything on the planet to eat right now—without any judgment about the food's calorie, protein, or carbohydrate content. What would that be? No one needs to know. It's a private fantasy.

3. Now think of the amount of this food you would love to have. Again, don't bring judgment to your decision. How much would you really like to have? Imagine you can see the food and the amount you just visualized. It's just there in front of you. Is it in a serving dish? On a plate?

4. Now you've eaten the food. Imagine this food is now in your stomach. How does it feel? Does the amount feel just right? Too much? Is it pushing on your stomach? Is it making you feel bloated? Does your stomach hurt?

5. Ask your body how much would be okay to eat so you feel comfortably full, alert, and energized.

6. Now imagine this food is moving down into your digestive system. Ask your body how the food feels in your digestive tract. Is there any discomfort in that part of your body as the food is being digested, such as pain, bloating, or gas?

7. Ask your body how much of this food would be okay to eat for you to feel good. Then modify the amount you ate to fit the "feel good" amount, meaning that any symptoms of dis—comfort are gone.

8. Now imagine the food has been digested. The nutrients are being absorbed into your bloodstream, and they're circulating through the brain, through the muscles, the organs, the skin; all your cell tissues are now being nourished.

9. After envisioning the optimal amount of food you can eat and still feel comfortable, scan your body to see whether there are any changes in sensations or feelings.

Give Yourself Permission to Eat

Whether your hunger is physical or symbolic, if you really want to eat a cookie, that's what you ought to do: eat the cookie without judging yourself. A key reason people overeat is that they impose restrictions on themselves about what they should eat, and then they don't eat what they really want. When you do this, you continue to "chase" whatever you were trying to get from the cookie.

Birsinger believes you won't overeat if you practice the mind—body visualization "because we're born with this ability to 'know' what and how much to eat," and the guided imagery technique is a way to reconnect to this. For instance, let's say you want a banana split, with whipped cream and hot fudge. But when you do the exercise, you realize the entire banana split is way too much for you to eat if you're to continue to feel comfortable in your body. When this hap—

pens, decide on the amount that'll feel good in your body, which may be only a couple of bites. Or not.

Birsinger offers this insight: if you don't do the guided imagery visualization described above, you're more likely to sit down and eat the whole banana split; you'll overeat and then feel stuffed. Self–sabotage may take over: "Now I've really blown it. That was way too much," you might think, but this only leads to more eating later, because you're likely to eat to berate yourself. And then, to feel better, you're going to have to eat again, and then restrict yourself, and then exercise, and then, on the rebound, overeat again—and so on. "All this happens because you've lost touch with your internal cues of what, when, and how much to eat," Birsinger says. "But when you make the connection to how much you need to feel okay, your mind–body remembers it. And then you—not food—are in charge of your emotions."

Transform the Craving

Here's another technique Birsinger created to help transform nega–tive, unpleasant feelings that lead to emotional eating into pleasant, sense–filled emotions that fill without food:

- Using all your senses, find ways to evoke the feeling you get doing an enjoyable activity (such as yoga or meditation or taking a walk). Have a something nearby that represents the pleasur–able activity—for example, a picture of a beautiful seascape, a heart–shaped paperweight, a lucky coin. Choose anything you like as a symbol to represent the activity.

- What do you love about the particular activity? If it's a walk on the beach, do you love the sound of the ocean? The air? Putting your feet in the sand?

- Find a fragrance you love. Cinnamon? Vanilla? Musk? To trans–form your craving, inhale your favorite scent. By doing so, you're symbolically filling up your senses with your favorite activity. You can also try this with textures, sounds, and so on.

Fill your senses as much as possible with the scent until you can evoke the feeling you get when you're actually doing your activity of choice. Enjoy the journey instead of food.[10]

Fine-Tuning Feelings with Food

There's yet another way you can take charge of emotional eating. Replace unpleasant feelings that drive you to overeat with conscious food choices that hold the power to enhance your mood. The following scenario will give you an idea about how you can fine-tune your feelings to your advantage.[11]

Susan is often overwhelmed with all-day fatigue, minimal motivation, and a sluggish metabolism. Her sister, Allison, feels edgy, irritable, and nervous, symptoms that worsen because of bouts of indigestion that make it hard for her to fall or stay asleep. Their dad, Tom, who has always been a competent accountant, more and more often has memory lapses and trouble recalling information. Their mom is dealing with the same old symptoms: constant cravings for carbohydrates, feeling blue and bloated, and depression about her stubborn weight gain.

Be balanced. Susan, Allison, and their parents are unaware that natural "chemical messengers" released from the foods they choose can modify their moods, alleviate anxiety, bolster brain power—even curb the urge to splurge on that donut. Therefore they continue to consume their "routine cuisine." They aren't alone in their ignorance of four key neurotransmitters—*dopamine, acetylcholine, gamma-aminobutyric acid* (GABA), and *serotonin*—that influence everything from energy and mood to memory and metabolism. When these four hormones are in balance, your mind-body is poised for peak performance. But when a dip in one or more causes an imbalance, symptoms can range from fatigue and weight gain to confusion and depression.

Balancing Rx: But there's good news: You can choose "designer foods" that reduce unpleasant feelings and unwelcome behaviors. Instead of feeding that drive to overeat, food can serve as your anti-emotional eating ally with the power to bring emotional balance, enhance energy, alleviate anxiety, and contribute to clearer thinking.

Instead of caving into cravings, you can put yourself in the driver's seat and take your feelings where you want them to go.

Enhance energy. Do you ever feel fatigue or lethargy throughout the day, even after a full night's sleep? If low energy is typical for you, the cause could be dopamine deficiency. From fabulous flavors to sensual scents, if your brain interprets a food (or an activity) as pleasurable and you tend to turn to it for a pleasure hit, it may be because you're seeking the feel-good response of dopamine. In essence, dopamine works its wonders by stimulating the central nervous system (CNS), keeping energy levels, motivation, and excitement high.

Dopamine Rx: The pleasure-producing ingredients in high-protein foods are the amino acids tyrosine and phenylalanine, building blocks of both protein and dopamine. To elevate mood and energy, consider consuming water-packed tuna, low-fat yogurt, or lean meat.

Alleviate anxiety. If anxiety, nervousness, and irritability—with bouts of indigestion and trouble sleeping—are all too familiar, it may mean you have low levels of GABA. A nerve chemical and nerve modulator that stimulates the central nervous system, this natural sedative works its wonders by controlling brainwave rhythms, which in turn regulate behavior.

GABA Rx: Produce more GABA by choosing foods high in the B vitamins, especially B_6. How B_6 affects the nervous system and brain isn't completely understood, but even marginal intakes influence levels of GABA and other mood-modifying neurotransmitters. Boost dietary intake of this B vitamin with whole grains, dark leafy greens, bananas, avocados, and protein-rich chicken, fish, legumes, and nuts.

Defog. Some older people call it a "senior moment"; others who find it harder and harder to recall information might say they're experiencing a memory lapse. Those who study food and mood may interpret such symptoms of "brain fog" to be a sign of acetylcholine deficiency. Produced in the brain by the fatlike substance *choline*, this nerve chemical is a building block of *myelin*, which helps CNS cells communicate.

Acetylcholine Rx: To manage general mental functioning, boost brain levels of this memory manager by consuming choline−rich foods such as wheat germ, fish, eggs, blueberries, and peanuts, all of which are converted into acetylcholine during digestion.

Curtail cravings. Do you crave high−carbohydrate, high−salt foods such as cookies, cake, and chips—especially when you're feeling blue? Do you feel hungry even when you're full? Is weight gain a constant? If so, your supply of serotonin may be low. Soothing serotonin is a natural antidepressant; it also contributes to stable blood sugar levels, which in turn prevent food cravings and the urge to overeat.

Serotonin Rx: To produce more serotonin, seek out foods rich in the amino acid tryptophan, such as avocado, poultry, and wheat germ, or foods high in complex carbohydrates, such as potatoes (with the skin), beans, and whole grains.

Instead of feeding that drive to overeat, food can serve as your anti−emotional eating ally with its power to bring emotional balance, enhance your energy, alleviate anxiety, and contribute to clearer thinking. Instead of caving into cravings, put yourself in the driver's seat and take your feelings where you want them to go.

"B" Wise

From dreary doldrums to a deeper depression, various B vitamins—including B_1, B_2, niacin, folic acid, and B_{12}—can help you bust the blues. To help defeat depression, "B" wise and consider the following guidelines when deciding which foods to eat.

Choose whole foods. Fast food "is a loser when it comes to vitamins and minerals that help to boost spirit," writes nutritionist Elizabeth Somer. Folic acid in particular (the most common nutritional deficiency in the United States) is linked to depression, as are other B−family relatives that are processed out of refined foods: B_6, niacin, and B_{12}. Some especially good B−abundant blues busters are unprocessed, unrefined grains (whole wheat, oats, millet, brown rice, etc.), fruits, vegetables, beans, nuts, and seeds. Vitamin B−rich greens such as spinach are especially good for this.

Shake the sugar habit. Consuming a lot of refined white sugar both damages and destroys B vitamins in the body; in this way, it contributes to deficiencies. Eliminate sugar from the diet, and depression often lifts—although why this is so isn't well understood. One theory is that the "high" a person derives from sugar is due to elevated glucose (blood sugar) and endorphins, which produce feelings of relaxation and euphoria. When the sugar in food is metabolized, blood sugar levels along with endorphins and other hormones "crash," contributing to depression and fatigue. When a diet is rich in foods loaded with vitamin B and low in sugar, the levels of B vitamins, glucose, and endorphins remain stable, reducing the chances of depression.

Avoid or limit alcohol and caffeine. Consuming too much alcohol and caffeine can cause the loss of certain B vitamins—and deficiencies of vitamins B_6 and niacin, especially, can bring you down. Not only does excessive alcohol and caffeine consumption reduce the absorption of B vitamins, but it also contributes to protein and mineral deficiencies.[12]

Many of us have felt sad or have had the Monday morning blahs at times; others—more than fifteen million Americans—experience serious depression during their lifetime. Include more foods high in the B vitamins, and you may improve your mood and be less likely to experience depression linked to emotional eating.

Access Your Appetite

The science that studies nutrients in the foods we consume, and the way they influence our brain chemistry and emotions, provides a peek into how food and the mind and body work together. By being aware of whether you "feel" like eating to appease a healthy appetite, each food you choose to eat may be looked at as an opportunity not only to feed your body but also to fine-tune your moods and emotions. Here's the prescription for overcoming emotional eating and choosing instead to eat when your mind-body is ready to "welcome" food and anticipate it for the pleasure it will bring:

Emotional Eating Rx: Eat for pleasure—when you have an appetite and you're experiencing feel-good feelings.

In other words, the key to success is making a commitment to eating for pleasure—when you have a healthy, authentic appetite for food and you're anticipating the pleasure of eating.

Chapter 5

Get Fresh

One evening after physician Mark A. Hyman had given a lecture, a sixty–year–old morbidly obese man named Samuel approached him. Weighing more than 300 pounds, Samuel asked Hyman if he would be his doctor. Hyman agreed.

During the office visit, Samuel described a life filled with excessive overeating and bingeing; for instance, two cups of heavy whipping cream each night was a typical nightcap. He had a history of extreme yo–yo dieting: losing weight and then gaining it back . . . plus even more. As his obesity worsened, so did his health. By the time Samuel came to see Hyman, he had a plethora of infirmities— profound fatigue, difficulty breathing while walking, stuffed sinuses, swollen legs, severe sleep apnea, dry skin, imbalanced hormones, food sensitivities, and an impaired liver—as well as a wide range of risk factors linked to heart disease, such as diabetes.

What happened next changed Samuel's health and weight, indeed his life, forever. Hyman gave him hope. "I told him that if he did everything I suggested, he would lose weight, feel better, and his symptoms would go away. Everything he had done, he did to himself and could undo," writes Hyman.

What did Hyman suggest? The core of the program he recommended was a diet abundant in nutrient–dense, fresh, unprocessed whole foods (fruits, vegetables, whole grains, beans and peas, and nuts and seeds) "without any restriction on calories or portion size." To enhance Samuel's weight loss, Hyman included a conservative exercise plan of walking slowly, then added interval training once Samuel was in better shape. He also augmented Samuel's fresh food diet and exercise plan with supplements and herbs that would be helpful in turning around his various ailments. Armed with this advice, Samuel left Hyman's office somewhat skeptical but determined.

After three months on the program, Samuel had lost thirty pounds, his food cravings had disappeared, and some of his symptoms were less severe. Eight months later, "I was shocked when he weighed in," writes Hyman. "He had lost 110 pounds without being on a strict deprivation diet." There was more good news: along with his excess weight, most of Samuel's ailments had vanished or diminished. Just as encouraging, having replaced a diet of mostly fast, processed, fat−filled food with fresh, whole, flavor−filled nourishment, what remained was his "continued pleasure in food," writes Hyman. Samuel achieved weight and health success—without deprivation, without restricting calories, and without suffering—in large part because he replaced a predominantly high−calorie, empty−calorie, fast−food diet with a low−fat, nutrient−dense, fresh, and whole−food way of eating that provided the nutrients—in the ratio nature intended—that his body needed to heal.[1]

What was it about Samuel's change from fast food to a fresh−, whole−food way of eating that led to such powerful—seemingly effortless—improvements in his weight and well−being? And if it worked for him, might it be beneficial for the millions of us who struggle with the perennial weight loss question: what's the best diet for losing weight and keeping it off? A look at the fast foodism eating style can give us clues about how a diet of mostly fast and processed foods increases your likelihood of being overweight—and, in con−trast, how consuming mostly fresh, whole foods—as Samuel did—can lead to weight loss that often is effortless.

Foodish Food

Some say it's "snack crack." Others imply it's an "industrial artifact," while corporations call it a "commodity." Our friend and colleague, naturopathic physician Bruce Milliman, calls it "ersatz food," meaning that it's "an inferior substitute imitating an original." The Center for Science in the Public Interest (CSPI) calls it "food porn." We call it "foodish food"—the opposite of the fresh, whole, lean food that helped Samuel lose weight.

Foodish food typically has three characteristic attributes: it is fast, processed, and unhealthy. Most everyone is familiar with fast food, which is inexpensive and prepared and served quickly in restaurants such as McDonald's, Burger King, Wendy's, KFC, and Taco Bell.[2] Processed food, on the other hand, has been cooked, baked, cured, heated, dried, mixed, ground, separated, extracted, sliced, preserved, dehydrated, frozen. Because processed food is often manufactured, it's typically packaged, canned, jarred, or enclosed in some other sort of container.[3] Fast and processed foods have one thing in common: both are junk food, a slang term referring to fare that's high in calories, salt, sugar, fat, and additives but low in nutrients such as fiber, vitamins, and minerals—hence the term "empty calories."[4]

Foodish food—open the newspaper on any given day and you're likely to find it reviled as the scourge of the twenty−first century. As we write, we're scanning the following headlines: "It's a fat, fat, fat, fat world: America's blueprint for poor eating is being spread around the planet"; "Junk−food makers face FTC scrutiny: with childhood obe−sity rates rising, a group of food companies could be forced to disclose details on marketing to feds"; and "Sugar coated: We're drowning in high fructose corn syrup: do the risks go beyond our waistline?"[5]

What does the fast foodism eating style look like? A breakfast bar for breakfast; Chicken McNuggets with a Coke for lunch; and per−haps a pepperoni and sausage pizza, delivered from your nearby pizza parlor, for dinner. Add several soft drinks sipped throughout the day and some snacks of chips or cookies, and you have a profile of the typical cuisine for many Americans. Not surprisingly, this eating style is strongly linked with overeating and being overweight. And if you're a "fast fooder," you're at increased risk for heart disease, diabetes, high blood pressure, certain cancers, and other ailments—meaning that fast foodism threatens more than your waistline.

Toxic Food Environment
Psychologist Kelly Brownell, co−founder and director of the Rudd Center for Food Policy & Obesity at Yale University, is a leading

obesity expert. And he links the obesity epidemic in America in large part to the "toxic food environment" that the fast–food industry has created. According to Brownell, this ranges from easy access to foodish foods to an excess of advertising.

"We take Joe Camel off the billboard because it is marketing bad products to our children, but Ronald McDonald is considered cute. How different are they in their impact?" asks Brownell, meaning that both cigarette smoking and excess consumption of fast foods are health threats.[6] Add the supersizing of such fast–food staples as burgers, franks, fries, and other foods that are already high–calorie and super–processed—foods often laden with trans fats, sugar, and refined flour—and the alarming increase in obesity should hardly come as a surprise.

With Americans spending 40 percent of their food budget on restaurant meals, compared to 25 percent in 1970, many are indeed living the fast foodism eating style that's contributing to our growing girth. A closer look at the ingredients often added to fast foods will give you a better understanding of why we believe fast food isn't really food in the traditional sense—it's foodish food, ersatz sort–of–like–food food, but not real food—and why the modifications that make it, well, fast food can contribute to your growing girth.

Take-Aways, Add-Ins

The health–robbing problem with fast food is twofold: what fast food manufacturers process out of food, and what they add.

Take-aways. In the 1750s in England, the invention of machinery used in manufacturing changed the way we make food forever. It was the roller mill, especially—huge cylinders that could crush and separate the wheat kernel into its elements of flour, germ, and bran—that made the difference. More than a century later, porcelain mills enabled manufacturers to make white flour—in lieu of whole–wheat flour—inexpensively; ergo, white flour became a popular, easily avail–able staple for the masses. It was called "separated food" because the mill separated the bran, germ, and endosperm (flour) elements of the wheat kernel.

Today we call white flour "refined" or "processed." The health-enhancing "good" fats, vitamins, minerals, antioxidants (that protect body cells from the damaging effects of oxidation), and phytochemicals (naturally occurring substances in plant-based foods that have beneficial health effects) have been processed out of the whole kernel. It has also been refined to have a long shelf life and be easy to use as an ingredient of baked goods.

Add-ins. When wheat was being denatured, nutritional science as we know it didn't exist. In the eighteenth century, French chemist Antoine-Laurent Lavoisier had defined the *calorie*, a measure of energy in food, and then in the 1840s German scientist Justus von Liebig isolated proteins, fats, carbohydrates, and minerals in food. But these discoveries were just that—discoveries.

Nothing much changed in the nutrition world until the early 1900s, when diseases of malnutrition such as beriberi and pellagra began to among populations who were consuming separated grains: in England and America, where white flour was popular, and in Japan and China, where the population had turned from brown rice to milled, processed, denatured white rice. To combat widespread malnutrition, food manufacturers enriched (added back to) white flour and white rice products the four nutrients we then knew about that had been lost in processing: niacin, riboflavin, thiamin, and iron. This enrichment didn't include fiber or the germ or the more than twenty-five vitamins and minerals we know about now.

Today, to compensate for what's missing, most of the food made by the multibillion-dollar fast-food industry contains more than a few added vitamins and minerals in white-flour products (such as hamburger buns). To standardize flavor, mouth feel, and sense of satiety, fat and sugar also have become typical additions—increasing calories.

While fast food alone isn't causing obesity rates to soar (eating habits, physical activity, genetics, and lifestyle all play a part), in country after country that adopts American eating habits—including lots of foodish food—obesity increases dramatically. Consider France, where childhood obesity increased steadily for decades due to the adoption of lifestyle habits such as more fast food and less physical activity.

What's especially telling (and hopeful), though, is that by 2008—unlike other European countries with *increasing* obesity rates—the trend toward childhood obesity in France had stabilized due to effective governmental policies that promote a healthier diet. A closer look at ingredients added to fast foods gives some clues about why they can put you on the fat track.

Four Weight Boosters in Fast Food

From fried fish and fries to hamburgers and pizza, the food served in restaurants such as McDonald's, Denny's, and Pizza Hut is familiar to most of us. What may be less well known is that the food is highly processed, prepared in bulk at industrialized central locations, and then shipped to each restaurant.

It's during the processing that a seemingly simple item, say white flour–based buns, becomes high–calorie, high–fat, sugar–laden foodish food. Not only is lots of fat and sugar added, but the *type* of fat that's often used—partially hydrogenated oil—is so toxic to your health and waistline that some places, including New York City, have banned its use in restaurants. And then there are all those highly processed sweeteners that wreak havoc with your weight.

Researcher Robert Lustig, professor of pediatrics at UCSF (University of California, San Francisco) Children's Hospital, describes the fast–food "fat–track problem" this way: "Our current Western food environment has become highly 'insulinogenic,' as demonstrated by its increased energy density (caloric intake), high fat content, high glycemic index, increased fructose composition, [and] decreased fiber . . . ." After conducting a large–scale review (called a meta–analysis) of obesity research, Lustig concluded that too much processed fructose (a type of sugar) and not enough fiber "appear to be cornerstones of the obesity epidemic through their effects on insulin."[7]

To give you a sense of the problematic ingredients *added* to fast food that pose serious health problems, let's take a closer look at the recipe for a regular McDonald's hamburger bun. Here are the ingredients in a McDonald's bun, listed according to quantity from most to least:

Enriched bleached flour (bleached wheat flour, malted barley flour, thiamine, riboflavin, niacin, folic acid, reduced iron), water, high fructose corn syrup, partially hydrogenated soybean oil, yeast, con—tains less than 2 percent of each of the following: salt, calcium sul—fate, calcium carbonate, calcium silicate, wheat gluten, soy flour, baking soda, emulsifier (mono— and diglycerides, diacetyl tartaric acid esters of fatty acids, ethanol, sorbitol, polysorbate 20, potassium propionate), sodium stearoyl lactylate, dough conditioner (corn—starch, ammonium chloride, ammonium sulfate, calcium peroxide, ascorbic acid, azodicarbonamide, enzymes), calcium propionate (preservative). Contains wheat and soybean ingredients.[8]

The unfamiliar ingredients on the list may seem daunting, but it's the three "silent killers," abundant in many fast foods, which warrant your attention and concern: white flour, high fructose corn syrup, and partially hydrogenated oil.

Enriched bleached flour. We've explained that enriched flour is made by first separating the three original elements of the wheat kernel—flour, germ, and bran, or outer shell. The life—giving nutri—ents found in the germ (which has all eight B vitamins and healing substances called *phytochemicals*), the naturally occurring nutrients in the bran (mostly fiber and B vitamins) itself are removed. What's left is the white flour, the *endosperm* part of the kernel, which consists mostly of carbohydrates and protein along with an unbalanced ratio of macronutrients (fat, carbohydrates, protein) and micronutrients (vitamins and minerals).

Denatured white flour together with no fiber to slow down the absorption of food creates a formula for making and retaining fat. Consume lots of white—flour products and you increase your chances of gaining weight, because these foods are absorbed quickly by your body. Levels of glucose (sugar) and insulin (a hormone or "chemical messenger") rise, along with the amount of circulating fat.

High fructose corn syrup. "Sugar: the ingredient you can trust. And pronounce. There's just one ingredient in real, all—natural sugar:

real, all–natural sugar. Plus, it's only 15 little calories per teaspoon. And that's all there is to it."[9] This ad by the sugar industry recently ran in my local newspaper. Is it accurate? Absolutely. At the same time, though, it hides the whole story: what's hidden is the powerful place sugar takes in the creation of fast, processed foods. Call it sugar, sucrose, fructose, maple syrup, molasses, dextrose, turbinado, amazake, sorbitol, carob powder, or high fructose corn syrup—it's sugar. And it's there in most fast foods—abundantly.

We chose as an example of fast food a seemingly innocuous hamburger bun because, unlike a donut, most of us don't think of a bun as having a lot of sugar, fat, or calories. But the carbohydrate content (sugar is carbohydrate–dense) of a McDonald's hamburger is thirty–seven grams. Since meat doesn't have any carbohydrates (it's composed of protein, fat, vitamins, and minerals), this means that the bun, by itself, is contributing the carbohydrates—mostly from white flour and added sugar.

The ad from the sugar industry said that one teaspoon of sugar is "only 15 little calories per teaspoon. And that's all there is to it." But that's not all there is to it—not when a hamburger bun, which isn't even known for being a sweet, has more than 135 calories, much of which is from sugar alone! And the fact that the sweetener is in the form of high fructose corn syrup (HFCS) really raises a health alarm—as well as a notch on your belt. Why? When you consume the fructose (a form of sugar that comes from fruit) in the super–processed HFCS added to thousands of fast foods and beverages, your brain doesn't recognize that it's a food, or that it has calories (energy)—although it is, indeed, calorie–dense. Instead, your brain thinks you're starving; to compensate, it signals you to keep eating. In other words, HFCS ignites your hunger signals, and though you're consuming lots of calories, you're still hungry. In response, you eat more . . . and gain more weight.[10]

Partially hydrogenated oil. Unlike naturally occurring poly–unsaturated, monounsaturated, and saturated fats in food, partially hydrogenated oil is artificially created from plant–based foods—fruit, vegetables, grains, beans and peas (legumes), and nuts and seeds. Food manufacturers pump hydrogen atoms into liquid oils (making them "partially hydrogenated") in order to thicken them, enhance flavor, and increase the shelf life of foods that contain them.

Hydrogenation changes the molecular structure of the oil, which in turn decreases rancidity (decomposing and becoming stale). Examples of food products that have been partially saturated with hydrogen atoms include some spreadable, soft margarines and vegetable shortening. When a food or oil is completely—rather than partially—saturated with hydrogen atoms, the result is hard, firm fat, the kind you see in chilled bacon, beef, or butter.

So what's the problem? Why have New York and other cities banned food prepared with partially hydrogenated oils in their restaurants? Partial hydrogenation process creates *trans fatty acids*, commonly called *trans fat*. Unlike naturally occurring polyunsaturated and monounsaturated fats, artificially made trans fats pose serious health risks—heart disease, type 2 diabetes, obesity. The siren has been sounded against trans fats—loudly—by health professionals nationwide, in Canada, and throughout Europe. The consensus: trans fat isn't safe. If you consume foods containing trans fat, you should keep your intake to one gram or less.[11] Look at labels. As of January 2006, trans fat is listed along with saturated fat and cholesterol on the Nutrition Facts label of packaged foods in this country.

To decrease body fat, one of the best actions you can take is to avoid any food that lists partially hydrogenated oil as an ingredient, because *trans fat makes you fatter than other fats do*. Researchers at Wake Forest University fed the same number of calories to monkeys over a six-year period, with 8 percent of one group's calories coming from olive oil (which is mostly monounsaturated fat) and 8 percent of a second group's calories coming from industrially made trans fat. The monkeys who ate the trans fats gained four times more weight than those on the olive oil–based diet. The main fast-food culprits containing trans fats: fried and baked food products.

Calories. Denatured white flour, high fructose corn syrup, and trans fats are key players when it comes to putting on pounds, but *the* major player, unequivocally, is the number of sugar and fat calories in the supersized portions offered in our nation's 300,000 fast–food res–taurants. The arithmetic is easy: large portions equal large waistlines.

Due to supersizing and the added sugar and fat, fast–food afi–cionados consume about 200 calories more each day than they did a decade ago. This may not seem like much, but it could mean a gain of five pounds each year; kids can put on six pounds a year from fast food. Consider a sample meal from McDonald's: a Big Mac sandwich (7.8 ounces) has 560 calories, a medium serving of French fries (4 ounces) is 380 calories, and a medium Coca–Cola (21 ounces) comes to 210 calories. Total calories in one meal: 1150.[12]

Clearly, the ingredients in fast food and Americans' love affair with this foodish food have created a deep and multidimensional problem in the United States. Though a diet of mostly foodish food plays havoc with our health and weight, one–quarter of our adult population visits a fast–food restaurant on any given day. We are, indeed, a fast–food nation.

There's a simple way to eat that provides the antidote to fast foodism. It's a time– and science–tested guideline that has nourished humankind for millennia—and it's how people who are naturally thin eat today. The secret of eating to get slim and stay slim lies in four simple words: fresh, whole, lean food—the dietary advice that phy–sician Mark Hyman gave to his obese patient Samuel. By following this general guideline, Samuel was able to lose 110 pounds without eating–by–number: calorie–counting, weight watching, counting carbs. It worked for him, and it can work for you.

Inverse Eating

You've heard it before: you should eat five or more serving of fruits and vegetables every day. But though Uncle Sam's dietary recommen–dations have been touted on TV and in newspapers nationwide, less than half of Americans (46.6 percent) manage to do this. Why are such seemingly simple dietary guidelines so hard for so many of us to follow?

In our opinion, simply put, that's just not the way most Americans eat. Our daily diets more typically include food from the animal–based food groups of dairy, poultry, meat, and fish. Not only do we eat a lot of these foods, but we often eat them in a fast and processed form: dairy in the form of ice cream; chicken that's been fried (some–

times served abundantly in buckets); processed meats such as salami, bacon, and ham; and canned tuna "marinated" in added oil and salt.

On the other side of the food–group spectrum are the plant–based food groups that typically *don't* make it to the American table: fruits, vegetables, whole grains (such as brown rice, oats, barley, whole wheat, and quinoa), legumes (beans and peas), and nuts and seeds. Before we tell you about the slimming secrets of plant–based foods (hint: there's more to it than fewer calories) and lean, fresh animal–based foods, you'll get the most from this chapter if you understand this basic con–cept: fruits, vegetables, whole grains, legumes, and nuts and seeds are the only naturally occurring plant–based food groups; dairy (such as milk, cheese, and yogurt), eggs, poultry, meat (both red and white, such as beef and pork), and fish are the only animal–based food groups.

Most of us develop weight problems because typical American fare focuses on foods that aren't fresh, whole, and lean; they're highly processed, packaged foods replete with calories, health–harming fat, denatured white flour, and sugar—salami instead of lean beef, or a donut or Danish instead of multigrain cereal with no added sugar. If plant–based foods are in our diet at all, they're likely to come in the form of French fries, baked goods (made with white flour and lots of added fat and sugar), or a sprinkling of lettuce (usually iceberg) that we flavor with bottled dressing high in fat, sugar, and calories.

In other words, we eat lots of *processed* dairy, poultry, meat, and fish, with smaller, occasional servings of denatured fruits, vegetables, grains, legumes, seeds, and roasted, salted, and fat–laden nuts (such as peanut butter with added trans fat). Often if we do choose whole–grain bread, a close look at the label reveals it's laden with unwanted additives such as HFCS or partially hydrogenated oil.

We use the term "inverse eating" to describe the *opposite* of how more and more Americans are eating. Inverse eating means a diet that consists mostly of fresh, whole, plant–based foods, supplemented—almost as if they were condiments—with small servings of fresh, lean, low–fat meat, poultry, fish, or dairy foods. For thousands of years, inverse eating has been the norm for most cultures—and their populations are thinner and healthier for it. Take the much–touted Mediterranean diet, for instance; the food eaten daily by people living in Greece, Italy,

Spain, and Portugal hasn't changed much in thousands of years. It still emphasizes fruits, vegetables, grains, and legumes, with low to moderate amounts of dairy, poultry, and fish. Small servings of red meat are occasional fare. In Greece, the fat comes mostly from fresh–pressed olive oil (no trans fat), feta cheese (naturally low–fat), and fresh yogurt.

Researchers from Cornell, Oxford, and Beijing universities were so intrigued by the inverse way of eating in China that they spent a decade studying the relationship between China's ancient diet and the health of its citizens. The China Project began in 1983 when scientists began analyzing the diets of 6,500 families in 130 rural villages not yet infiltrated by Western fast food. The data they collected and began to analyze in 1990 confirmed a diet based on grains (in the south) and corn, wheat, and millet (in the north); mineral–dense vegetables; and protein from soybeans and grains. Meat and other animal–based foods were eaten only occasionally and as condiments—seemingly to improve or adjust the flavor of a dish—except during special feasts.

The researchers discovered that the traditional, time–tested Chinese diet consisted of 75 percent calories from carbohydrates, 10 percent from protein (mostly from plant–based food), and 15 percent from fat. What a contrast to Americans' way of eating: an average of 45 to 50 percent calories from carbohydrates, 15 percent from protein (most of it from animal sources), and about 35 percent from fat.

While China was once considered to have one of the leanest populations worldwide, however, the influx of American fast food has taken its toll. Today, out of a total population of 1.35 billion, 38.5 percent of the 2010 population were overweight (up from 25 percent in 2002; and nearly 100 million people are obese, up from 18 million in 2005. In the United States, more than two–thirds of adults are overweight or obese. Sadly, children are catching up with the adults: for the first time in American history, children are expected to have shorter lives than their parents because of their ever–increasing weight.[13]

You become what you eat, and you weigh how you live. Your lifestyle—especially your relationship to food—is a key determinant of your weight. What health professionals nationwide would like you to do about this is to use the information discovered about nutrition and weight over the decades to start a personal revolution—to take a stand against foodish food and make fresh, whole, lean food and inverse eating your most–of–the–time way of eating. Please note that we use the expression "your most–of–the–time way of eating," because we're suggesting that you do this *as often as possible*—not as a regimented, restricted way of eating. When you do choose to have fast food or any other food that isn't fresh, whole, and lean—enjoy it!

Consider what might happen if you actually put inverse eating into action every day. How would you feel? How would you look? How would it influence your weight?

Eat More, Weigh Less

It really is possible to eat more and weigh less.[14] Doesn't such a suggestion go against everything we've ever learned about weight loss? Actually, what "eat more, weigh less" really means is that if you eat more of certain *types* of food instead of focusing on the *amount* of food you eat, you are likely to lose weight. Calories from fast food and calories from fresh, whole, lean food aren't the same.

Fruit. An apple a day may do more than keep the doctor away; it may keep you slim. When researchers from the State University of Rio De Janeiro in Brazil put two groups of women on a comparable–calorie diet, those who snacked on an apple lost more weight than those who munched on oatmeal cookies. Why might this be? With an 85 percent water content and lots of soluble fiber, apples are filling; they also keep blood sugar levels even, which cuts cravings and signals to your brain that you're full. And because apples are a fresh, whole food, they supply the nutrients you need in the ratio intended by nature.

Vegetables. Studies have linked abundant mixed salads with weight loss. By "abundant," we're referring to more than the typical iceberg lettuce and tomato duo that often passes for a salad. Rather, we're talking about a resplendent mix that might include lettuces, spinach, and arugula tossed with cherry tomatoes, chopped mushrooms, sliced cucumber, chopped red and green peppers, sliced avocado, beans, lean chicken or baked tofu, a sprinkling of chopped walnuts, grated cheese, and perhaps some raisins.

When researchers at Penn State University studied women who consumed a satisfying salad prior to eating pasta for lunch, they discovered that they ate less pasta than those who hadn't had salad. And there are other weight–loss benefits to both fruits and vegetables: they are the only source of vitamin C. A Purdue University study suggests that vitamin C may be a significant weight–loss aid, helping you to burn fat during physical activity. In fact, this study suggests that vitamin C is a key determinant of weight loss.

Whole grains. Since whole grains were first cultivated more than ten thousand years ago, they've been a boon to health. Recent research from Harvard University, published in the *American Journal of Clinical Nutrition*, reveals that they also prevent weight gain. In a twelve–year study conducted with more than 12,000 nurses ages thirty–eight to sixty–three, researchers found that those who ate the most whole–grain foods (such as oatmeal, popcorn, wheat germ, and multigrain breakfast cereal) weighed less than those who ate the least. The difference was quite significant: women in the high whole–grain group had a 49 percent lower risk of gaining weight.

Legumes. It's a fact. Including dried legumes such as pinto, navy, and lima beans in your diet (not green beans or soybeans) can help you lose weight. When Maurice Bennink, professor of nutrition at Michigan State University, reviewed a plethora of studies on beans published over a twenty–five–year period, he discovered compelling evidence that beans work their weight–loss wonders in three ways:

- Satiety—beans are rich in fiber, so you feel full.

- Sustained energy—beans have a very low glycemic index and thus glucose is released slowly into the bloodstream, so your blood sugar remains stable.

- Reduced odds of eating calorie−dense fast foods—consuming low−glycemic−index foods tends to lead to subsequent choices of low−glycemic−index foods.

Nuts and seeds. Although they look like nuts, taste like nuts, and crunch like nuts, technically peanuts are legumes. But because most of us relate to them as nuts, we're telling you about the weight−management potential of *fresh, raw, unroasted* peanuts here in the "nuts and seeds" category. We wouldn't call any kind of high−fat nut a weight−loss food, but large−population studies have linked their consumption to lower weight than for nonconsumers.

To test these results, Richard Mattes and his team in the Department of Foods and Nutrition at Purdue University studied three groups, each of which consumed 500 calories of peanuts daily for eight weeks. People in group one, who ate the peanuts without any dietary directions at all, gained an average of just 2.2 pounds; those in the second group, who added the peanuts to their usual diets, gained only one pound; and those in the third group, who were asked to follow a low−fat diet and substitute 500 calories of peanuts for 500 calories from other foods, maintained their weight.

The mechanism by which peanuts minimize weight gain or help us maintain weight isn't completely clear. What is theorized, though, is that peanuts may work by being super filling.

Dairy. At least one dairy food has been linked with lower weight: low−fat yogurt. When researchers at the University of Tennessee, Knoxville, put people on a twelve−week weight−loss program, those who consumed three servings of yogurt daily lost twice as much weight at those who didn't eat yogurt. The study's lead researcher, Michael B. Zemel, speculates that the metabolic reason for this is that the calcium in yogurt *combined with the bio-active compounds in yogurt* speeds up the fat−burning process, at the same time decreasing the production of fat.

Eggs. It was only a brief study, which makes it hard to draw conclusions, but there just might be something slimming about eggs. When researcher Nikhil Dhurandhar from Pennington Biomedical

Research Center in Baton Rouge, Louisiana, gave study participants two eggs for breakfast one day and bagels for breakfast another day, the daily calorie totals were 400 lower on the egg days.

A possible reason for the difference: it's likely that high–protein, low–fat eggs promote satiety more than processed, white–flour bagels. (Note: Because eggs are high in *dietary* cholesterol, they can raise your *blood* cholesterol levels. If you have heart disease, you may want to limit or avoid consumption of eggs.)

Fish. Like eggs, fish is high in protein and low in fat. And researchers at Sweden's Karolinska Institutet found that when people ate fish for lunch, they consumed 11 percent less for dinner than those fed a beef–based lunch containing the same number of calories. It may be that fish protein is especially filling, or, suggests lead researcher Saeedah Borzoei, it could be the rich flavor of fish that satisfies (more about food flavor in Chapter 8, "Feed the Senses"). Interestingly, steamed white fish (such as halibut) ranks number one as the most filling out of thirty–eight foods in the Australian Satiety Index.

A balance of nutrients. From bio–active compounds in yogurt to fiber in whole grains and apples, what fresh foods have in common is that their components add up to more than the sum of their parts. In other words, while scientists have isolated particular nutrients that are either health–enhancing or health–robbing, the key to optimal nourishment is not to pursue "parts" of foods by turning mostly to synthetic supplements for health and well–being. Nature is the best nutritionist possible: *consume fresh whole foods in their natural state as often as possible*, and you'll obtain nutrients in the ratio nature intended.

The ingredients in fresh, whole, lean foods—many that we know about, and others that remain to be discovered—not only balance your weight and keep you lean, but also help prevent, treat, and reverse a plethora of ailments, from heart disease and diabetes to high blood pressure, cataracts, and arthritis. You receive many benefits when you inversely consume food that's as close to its natural state as possible, because fresh, whole, lean foods have the whole package of nutrients needed for optimal health and well–being.[15]

Get Fresh

Throughout this chapter, we've talked about the ways in which foodish food can make you fat and, in contrast, how fresh foods can lead to leanness—and a lifetime of delicious dining. Here's the anti-dote to fast foodism—replacing a diet of foodish food with real food on which body, mind, and soul can thrive:

Fast Foodism Rx: Choose fresh, whole food in its natural state as often as possible.

Fresh, whole foods can also be the solution to the other overeating styles. They are truly satisfying, so you're less likely to overeat. They contain nutrients that enhance emotions. And they are filled with flavor, making it easier to eat mindfully.

Chapter 6
Enjoy Food with Others

One of our most memorable meals wasn't an actual meal; it was a dining experience cradled in hospitality, friendship, and fresh, simple food.

The place: the patio of a friend's villa in a medieval town in Switzerland. The time: nearing midnight. The setting: like a Turner painting, an almost−full moon lighting the nearby lake. The food: an assortment of Italian cheeses, apples and oranges, and rich red wine. The social ingredients: the two of us, friends, and our hostess, Frau Bucher. As the evening evolved, so too did our sense of satisfaction, for at intervals throughout the evening each person made a spon−taneous toast, linking our hearts and souls and flavoring the food—indeed, the entire evening—with love.

Since then, we'd thought often about how we might imbue our meals with the same soul−satisfying ambiance that permeated that evening. Somehow, the thought wouldn't go away.

Perhaps it was divine intervention. Or fate, or similar sensibilities. We were gifted with the answer to our quest one New Year's Eve, when we met Nailia Menne at our friend Roslyn Layton's home. Originally from Kazakhstan, Nailia told us about the *tamada* tradition when we mentioned that the English language needed a new word to describe the invisible ingredients that had created the "meal magic" we'd experienced that moonlit night in Switzerland.

"There is an ancient tradition that no Kazakh celebration is com−plete without wine and a *tamada*, the host or toastmaster whose role is to create a pleasurable ambiance and ensure that everyone present is honored and enjoys the occasion," Nailia told us. "Whether the gathering is small or a meal for many, it is a great honor for the person who is asked to be the tamada. Throughout the meal, starting with the elderly for whom there is much respect, followed by those who have traveled far for the occasion, the tamada invites each guest to toast people, the food, or the event. From the first course to the main course and then dessert, the *tamada* invites a toast. In this way, every person is honored through the modern expression of an ancient tradition that embodies the best of friendship and shared food."

As New Year's Eve continued to unfold, we knew we had found not only the word but also a time–honored ritual that embodies the special spirit of that evening in Switzerland. And now we'd like to make a toast: this chapter is dedicated to tamada–flavored food and friendship . . . for everyone . . . all ways, all days.

Fare for One

We are a lonely culture, and nowhere is this more evident than in the millions who eat meals alone. While a tamada–flavored meal includes food and friendship and a welcoming and memorable dining experience for all, more often than not it's an eat–alone dining scene that plays out daily for millions of Americans. Children reach for a piece of packaged pizza, then eat it at the computer; single working women heat up their low–cal frozen meal in the microwave, then dine solo while watching TV; and anxious traveling salesmen are driven to dashboard dining while en route to yet another meeting.

Not surprisingly, these scenarios also reflect the other overeating styles: food fretting, task snacking, emotional eating, fast foodism, unappetizing atmosphere, and sensory disregard. After all, the seven eating styles are an interconnected family of eating behaviors that lead to weight problems.

Not only does our research shed light on the social isolation that often surrounds food and dining, but it also links it with the increased likelihood of being overweight. The more often people dine alone, we found, the higher their body mass index (BMI, the measure of body fat based on height and weight). In contrast, normal–weight people typically eat with others—and they are more likely to eat wholesome fresh food and less fast, processed food. This is a sobering observation, because it suggests that chronic social isolation while dining increases the probability that you'll not only overeat but also eat more of the kinds of food that can easily add pounds.

There is yet another way to look at solo dining: children, 'tweens, and teens who don't eat dinner with other family members are at high risk for supersizing themselves. The problem has so invaded our culture that Joseph A. Califano, Jr., founder and chairman emeritus of the National Center on Addiction and Substance Abuse at Columbia University and former U.S. Secretary of Health, Education, and Welfare, initiated "Family Day—A Day to Eat Dinner with Your Children" in 2001.[1]

For those who think that addiction and substance abuse have nothing to do with food and overeating, consider this: millions of Americans who overeat and zone out with fast food do, indeed, have a substance abuse problem. While they may not literally be addicted to food, they have a strong physiological or psychological depen—dency on food and a habit of overeating, which ultimately damages their weight and self—esteem.

Why are children and adolescents who don't eat meals with their families more prone to obesity? Some researchers have put this exact question to the test.

Family Fare

When Harvard University researcher Matthew Gillman looked at the eating habits of more than 16,000 boys and girls ages nine to four—teen, he discovered that those who usually or always ate dinner with their families were likely to consume more fruits and vegetables, less soda, and less fried, high—fat, and sugar—laden food. And we know from our eating styles research that fast, processed foods are strong predictors of weight gain. Gillman's study also revealed that while 43 percent ate dinner with their families every day, the older the child, the less often he or she was likely to share in the family meal.[2]

Richard Strauss, former director of the Childhood Weight Control Program (now called the "Pediatric Weight Control Program") at the Robert Wood Johnson Medical School in New Brunswick, New Jersey, is another academic who warns that not getting together at dinnertime is contributing to our epidemic of childhood obesity. With one in five American kids being overweight and still more suf-fering from obesity, the growing girth of adolescents has become an urgent national health problem. Of course, limited physical activity plays a part—the children in Strauss's study spent only twelve minutes a day doing hard, sustained exercise, while they spent up to five hours indoors playing video games and watching TV.[3] More threatening to health, though, is the typical consumption of large, high−fat food portions and sweet sodas. Merge inactivity with high−calorie meals eaten outside the home and you have a way of life that contributes to obesity and ensuing medical complications—hypertension, diabetes, high cholesterol, and orthopedic problems. A lifetime of low self−esteem is often part of the teenage obesity package.

With the health of our children at stake, Strauss firmly believes that the antidote is sharing family fare filled with fresh fruits, vegeta-bles, whole grains, legumes, and low−fat and lean dairy, fish, poultry, and meat—and increasing physical activity together (see Chapter 11, "Get Moving"). Strauss predicts, perhaps somewhat ominously, that without making fresh food and more activity a family affair, the obe−sity epidemic will continue.[3]

Social Ties

The idea that family meals can serve as a buffer against ailments emerged in a landmark twenty−five−year study that began in the early 1960s in the small town of Roseto, Pennsylvania, when a local physician told researcher Stewart Wolf that he rarely saw cases of heart disease in the town's Italian−American population. Intrigued, Wolf set out to study the Rosetans, hoping to discover why their rate of heart disease was so low. Even though they consumed a traditional high−fat, high−cholesterol Italian−American diet of sauces, sausages, and other artery−clogging food, the rate of heart disease and mor−tality from heart attacks remained low in Roseto.

As the long−term study progressed, so did the rate of heart dis−ease among the Italian−Americans—so much so that it soon equaled that of the general American population. When Wolf and his col−leagues scrutinized the data, the main difference that surfaced was the change in human relationships. When the study started, close family ties and community cohesion were the norm; it was common to find three generations living together in one home. But as the children became adults, they moved away from Roseto. Over time, family and community cohesion began to weaken, along with commitment to religion, relationships, and traditional values. The close–knit way of life that had united Rosetans since their migration to Roseto had first migrated to America in 1882 had ended—along with its prophylactic effect on heart disease.

Although the Roseto study explores the shift in heart disease of an Italian–American community over a quarter century, it is also about the influence of human relationships and social support on the metabolism of high–fat, high–cholesterol, calorie–dense foods. Amazingly, this study suggests that when social support is present in our lives, especially when we eat, *what* we eat is somehow metabo–lized differently. If social support can halt heart disease even when we consume foods perceived as *not* being heart healthy, might eating as a family influence whether or not we gain weight?[4]

Care-Filled Feeding

Research results on the people of Roseto seemed to have antici–pated future studies that would serendipitously link dining with others to health and healing benefits. Not too long after the Roseto study, researcher Robert M. Nerem at Emory University School of Medicine also discovered an invisible healing web connecting rela–tionships and the metabolism of potentially artery–clogging food. When Nerem set out to learn about the effect diet has on the devel–opment of coronary artery disease (CAD), a research assistant on his team fed high–cholesterol bits of rabbit chow to caged rabbits. When it was time to tally the results, team members were confounded: though all the rabbits were fed the same artery–clogging food, some of them had 60 percent less plaque (blockage) in their arteries.

Unable to understand why some rabbits showed early signs of heart disease and others didn't, Nerem and his team retraced each step of the study. Once again, the rabbits in the middle tier of cages fared better than those in the lower and higher rungs. Upon closer scrutiny, they realized that it was the rabbits in the middle that the research assistant would take out of their cages to hold, pet, talk to, and play with during feeding. It was harder for the petite assistant to reach the rabbits in the higher and lower tiers, but those in the middle received their food while being held.

Amazed, the scientists repeated the study under much more measured conditions. This time, some rabbits would be fed the high-cholesterol diet while being individually held on a regular basis, while those in the control group would be fed the same diet and be given normal laboratory animal care but wouldn't be personally nurtured while being fed. Again, the cared-for rabbits showed more than a 60 percent reduction in lesions compared to the comparison group, even though the serum cholesterol levels, heart rate, and blood pressure of all the rabbits were similar.[5]

Both the Roseto and the rabbit studies imply that there's a mystery to how we metabolize food, and that the consciousness we bring to meals matters. As physician Deepak Chopra said in describing just how powerful invisible nutrients such as social support can be to our well-being. "When you look at nutrition from a purely scientific point of view, there is no place for consciousness. And yet, consciousness could be one of the crucial determinants of the metabolism of food itself."[6]

These studies on the power of relationships and food metabolism suggest that social support impacts the way our bodies use our food—so much so that it has the power to halt the development of heart disease. Call it awareness, realization, or perception, the "consciousness" to which Chopra alludes implies a special sensibility—an invisible, hard-to-measure mystery—that somehow plays an essential and critical role in the metabolism of food itself. And when this consciousness is miraculously activated, not only can it neutralize potentially artery-clogging cholesterol and fat that we've consumed, but it also can protect us against disease.

Imagine! Without drugs or surgery or any special diet, you have the power to activate the mystery of consciousness and influence the way you metabolize food—and potentially your waistline and health—simply by dining in the company of others.

Resetting the American Table

Though the above studies suggest that many benefits await us when we turn a table for one into a feast for a few, eating alone is a way of life with which many of us are all too familiar. Americans are paying a big price for their often secluded, mindless munching, for what columnist and cookbook author Marion Cunningham, now in her nineties, has described as "a motel life"—going in, going out, then grabbing something to eat alone. "When you eat this way, you don't create deep connections," said Cunningham, "and you miss the opportunity to get to know about the people you're living with when you don't sit around the table and share yourself around food."

In the 1970s, aware of the trend of the disappearing family meal in America, the American Institute of Wine and Food created a group called Resetting the American Table. Its mission: urging parents to start cooking for their families. As a member of this group, national treasure Cunningham felt strongly about the need for what she called "social nourishment." As she told us, "We're fed more than food when we eat with others. Instead of taking a solitary trip through life, when you dine with family you learn to share and care for others, as well as social skills, tradition, and ritual. Talk begins to flow, feelings are expressed, and a sense of well-being takes over."[7] Such is the nour-ishment that beckons when we reset the American table.

Recipes for Social Satisfaction

When we're giving presentations and discussing social nutrition and the solo dining eating style, we often offer the following scenario for consideration.

Imagine it's wintertime at 6:30 PM and you're in your car, driving home from work. It's dark and cold outside, you're fairly hungry (if 1 is famished and 10 is stuffed, you're at level 3), and you won't be home for half an hour. As you drive in the rush-hour traffic, you're also feeling alone and isolated. But then you think about the meal that awaits you. You know that your grandmother, who lives with you, your spouse, and your three adolescent children, has been pre-paring dinner for the past few hours. You know that when you enter your home, your first greeting will be the aroma of her freshly made meal. As you hang up your coat, you'll glance at the dining table, set as always with for six; sighing with delight, you'll think about how welcoming it looks, and how lucky you are to come home to a homecooked meal with your family.

As you continue driving, somehow your reverie of what awaits you has kept your hunger in check. It's no longer gnawing at you, tempting you to stop at a fast–food outlet to get something—perhaps a muffin—to appease your appetite. Somehow, just the thought of the family meal has filled you enough that your hunger isn't setting off sirens of discomfort; instead, you realize that it's merely a signal that it's time for you to eat.

When we ask people to share their reaction to this scene, we often hear sighs of satisfaction, and comments such as "I feel peaceful," "I'm envious," or "I wouldn't fear my hunger and rush to fill it with fast food."

What follows are some recipes, literal and figurative, for starting your own social nutrition traditions—and for turning a table for one into a table for two, three, or more.

Set a Friendship-Flavored Table

In ancient Rome, after a three–course meal the host of the evening would ask guests to choose a *magister bibendi*, a toastmaster responsible for each person's alcohol consumption. This honored person would also select speakers for the evening and decide on topics for convivial conversation. Take your cue from both the ancient Romans and the tamada toast we told you about earlier to imbue your own meals with the same soul–satisfying connection to others.

When you're hosting a meal, ask one special guest to orchestrate the evening by creating a pleasurable atmosphere that ensures everyone is honored and enjoys the occasion. An easy way for the evening's *magister bibendi* to accomplish this is to invite each guest to toast people, the food, or the event—perhaps every fifteen minutes or so, starting with the first course and continuing through dessert. In this way, through the modern creative expression of an ancient tradition, you and your friends are creating your own ritual that encourages a welcoming and memorable meal for all. And now we'd like to make another toast: to "friendship–flavored" food.

Multigenerational Meal Memories

If there's one comment about her cooking that Anita Bellandi often made, it was, "No, it's not sauce, it's tomato *gravy*." Explains her grand-daughter, Vinita Azarow, "During a summertime job while in college, I lived with my Italian grandmother, *Nonna* Anita, in her flat in San Francisco's Marina district. When I arrived home for dinner, I would sometimes be greeted by the exquisitely familiar aroma of her tomato sauce. But ask my grandmother if she was making tomato sauce (*salsa di pomodoro*), and in her Italian accent she would often respond, 'No, I'm making tomato *gravy*.'"

While most of us would describe Nonna's elixir as sauce and not gravy, perhaps she had the original meaning of "gravy" in mind—for it initially signified a sort of spiced, stock-based sauce; only in the sixteenth century did its meaning as a "sauce made from meat juices" emerge.

More likely, the legacy of Nonna's tomato "gravy" has its roots in Italy, where various recipes evolved to form the bases of soups, stews, or sauces. Sometimes ingredients consist of *soffrito* (soh–FREE–toh), which literally means "under or barely fried" to describe finely minced carrots, celery, and onion that have been sautéed in olive oil. Optional additions include garlic, parsley, and a few leaves of fresh sage; if the recipe calls for it, *pancetta* (pan–CHEH–tuh), Italian bacon cured with salt, pepper, and other spices (but not smoked), may be included. Or another option might be *battuto* (bah–TOO–toh)—*soffrito* without the olive–oil sauté.

When we asked Vinita how she knew Nonna had made tomato gravy on certain days when she came home from work, her response was instant: "How do you describe that wonderful smell of the sauce cooking, the herbs, the basil, the garlic that went into it? There was a full flavor to it—not like prepared store–bought sauces that are overly tomato–y. Instead, Nonna's fresh ingredients and finely diced vegetables (some grown in her garden) created a rich underbase, a layering that was part of the complexity of the flavor."

Spicing the sauce with special social occasions added to its flavor. "Nonna would make and serve her special sauce during those times when the family would come over to her home," reflects Vinita. "The table would glow with her best crystal, china, and hand–embroidered linen tablecloth." Clearly, her granddaughter's summer−long stay also warranted serving the special sauce. "We would sit in her dining nook and eat the sauce with other fresh food she would cook for us. The meal was served on dishes with pink roses, not far from the kitchen door that led to the garden. It's still a special memory." [8]

As with the different generations of Italian−Americans in Roseto, Pennsylvania, eating a meal together seemed to make a difference in the well−being of Nonna's family. To create your own multigenera−tional memories:

- Start a family tradition by inviting one or more family mem−bers over to enjoy a meal made using a recipe from an older member of your family—perhaps an aunt or uncle, parent, or cousin. As Nonna did, set a glowing table with special ware.

- Create your own "family" by starting a cooking club. Invite coworkers, friends, and community members with whom you interact—a librarian, neighbors, people who work in restau−rants—to be part of your club. Rotate meals at the homes of members. In the spirit of tamada, share meal memories and stories as you dine.

- Make a favorite recipe and then invite friends and family from different generations to come for an informal meal.

- If you live alone, consider placing a picture of a family− or friendship−filled meal on the table as you eat. If your mother used to make a special meal that you particularly enjoyed, make it for yourself on a weekend and freeze it, then let it defrost while you're at work one day so you can enjoy it when you get home—reflecting on your family or friends as you eat.

- Prior to the latter half of the twentieth century, the recipes parents made for their families were often learned from *their* parents or other family members. Create your own culinary family tree and a connection to your roots, people— and food—wise, by putting together a collection of family recipes.

Nonna's Tomato Gravy

Recipe by Anita Giovacchini Bellandi and Vinita Bellandi Azarow

Make a simple meal of your favorite pasta mixed together with Nonna's tomato gravy, infused with the flavors of fresh, finely diced vegetables. Don't forget to sprinkle it with freshly grated cheese. "Nonna was partial to Pecorino Romano, but Parmesan is also good," Vinita says. "She always served the pasta with fresh greens dressed with red wine vinegar and extra—virgin olive oil, with salt and pepper to taste. San Pellegrino water would be on the table. And dessert might consist of an apple, with a couple of her anisette cookies."

"These amounts are approximate," says Vinita. "My Nonna didn't measure her ingredients. As I watched her, I guessed at the amounts she was using. Add or take away according to your taste."

1 to 2 tablespoons olive oil
1 small onion, finely chopped
1/2 stalk celery, finely chopped
1 small carrot, finely chopped
2 cloves garlic, finely chopped
1 tablespoon finely chopped fresh parsley
1 (28—ounce) jar plum tomatoes
4 to 6 basil leaves, torn into smallish pieces (if using dried basil, use ½ teaspoon and add it with the parsley)
Salt and pepper to taste
Sugar, as needed
2 tablespoons butter

To make the *soffrito*, heat the olive oil over medium heat. Lower the heat, then sauté the onion for 5 to 7 minutes, or until lightly golden. Add the celery, carrot, garlic, and parsley and cook for 5 more minutes, or until lightly browned. The garlic should turn a light golden color; be careful not to brown it. *(Note: Nonna often deglazed the vegetables by adding red wine and scraping up the browned bits before she added the plum tomatoes.)*

Decrease the heat to low. Break apart the plum tomatoes using your hands, then add them to the *soffrito*. Simmer about 5 minutes. Add the basil, and season with salt and pepper to taste. Add a bit of sugar to adjust the acidity of the tomatoes, if needed. Continue to simmer for about 20 minutes, or until the sauce has reached the desired thickness. When it's ready, the bubbles coming up will be a lighter orange color than the gravy. Just before serving, stir in the butter.

Variation: Tomato gravy with meat. Sometimes Nonna would make the tomato gravy with meat, Vinita says. "She would first brown a smashed clove of garlic in the olive oil and then remove it. Then she'd brown pieces of beef (ground beef, ground veal, or pieces of steak) in the garlic–flavored olive oil. At that point she'd remove the meat and deglaze the pan with a little wine (Marsala, or a good red that she had on hand). Then she would proceed to cook the vegetables as above, adding the meat back in during the final simmer."

Share Meaningful Meals . . . in Spirit

Ancient Romans followed pagan customs by feasting and eating to excess. Only the worship of their more moderate, frugal ancestors and their many gods served to curtail their gorging. Pagans believed that the gods depended on humans to create lodging for them in the form of temples and to nourish them through food offerings. Thinking that extravagant temples and abundant of food would keep the gods in a good mood, the Romans invited them to join in the meal. Only after the gods were offered the first mouthfuls of food and the first drops of wine did the Romans eat.

In the tradition of the ancient Romans, it is possible to share food with friends and family members—in spirit—even when dining alone. Just prior to eating, think of a family member, friend, or other person you admire, living or not. While thinking of this person—and perhaps also of a shared memory—place a small portion of your own food on a separate small plate next to your place setting. Add a drop or two of your beverage. Before eating, close your eyes and then inhale and exhale slowly as you reminiscence about your friend or family member. Throughout the meal, eat from your heart (see Chapter 8, "Feed the Senses") by continuing to reflect on the valued person.

Family Fare for the Twenty-First Century

Our friend Mary called one day to tell us about a new concept of family meals she'd just read about in our local newspaper. Knowing how time−pressured so many heads of household are, several women had gotten together to provide "everything you need to assemble delicious dinners for your family, store in the freezer, and then serve in the weeks ahead." All homemakers need to do is to call or stop by to order their meals, then pick up the fresh ingredients, already prepped, at their convenience. When they get home they assemble the ingredients and cook them. Voilà! Dinner is served.[9]

If such a service is a dream you don't think you can afford, or if it simply isn't available in your area, consider creating the same service for yourself by asking for assistance from family members or friends. Pick a day, set aside some time, and plan your meals for the week. Shop for ingredients and either assemble and prep them all in advance or, if you prefer, assemble and cook each meal independently as the need arises.

Enjoy Food with Others

The antidote to the solo dining eating style? Take a cue from Europeans, ancient Romans, and state−of−the−art science and share your food experiences with others—either literally or in spirit. As often as possible, enjoy a fresh meal or snack with coworkers, family, or friends. The solution looks like this:

Solo Dining Rx: Share food-related experiences with others.

As simple as the solution to the solo dining eating style may seem, we know it can be a challenge to implement, given the demands of busy schedules and cell phones, pagers, and e—mail that can keep us on call twenty—four hours a day. But you'll find the rewards well worth the effort.

Chapter 7

Dine by Design

Both the *psychological* and the *aesthetic* atmospheres in which you dine hold the power to influence your weight and well–being. What do we mean by psychological and aesthetic atmospheres? Have you ever eaten in an especially pleasant place, surrounded by supportive people, convivial conversation, and beautiful accoutrements? Perhaps friends took you to a welcoming restaurant for your birthday; because they'd organized the meal to celebrate you, the evening crackled with joy, conversation, and laughter.

The *external* mood, tone, and ambiance that surrounds you while you eat determines the psychological atmosphere. In the example of the birthday party, the atmosphere is celebratory and a source of pleasure. The milieu has an agreeable effect on you psychologically as you and your friends chat over a delicious meal. In response, your heart is open and your soul is singing.

But the psychological atmosphere can also be negative, stress–filled, and unpleasant. Have you ever eaten while being scolded or criticized? Or while driving during rush hour? Or while watching a horror movie or murder mystery on TV? If so, you've had the experience of eating in an unpleasant psychological atmosphere. The surroundings were so hectic or unpleasant that they affected your mind or mental processes in some way—either consciously (when you're being scolded while eating, for example) or unconsciously (you might not be aware of the impact a horror movie is having on your psyche or digestive process).

The other important component of the "unpleasant atmosphere" eating style is the aesthetics that surround you when you eat. Is the place in which you're dining welcoming in appearance? If you're sitting on a hard plastic bench, eating off damp paper plates on a garishly colored plastic tabletop, your dining aesthetics are less than optimal. Or perhaps you're eating on the run in a noisy fast–food restaurant with rock music blaring and fluorescent lighting glaring overhead. These are examples of aesthetically unpleasant surround–ings. (Of course, it's all in the eye of the beholder! The same aesthetics may be pleasing to some.)

As a contrast, envision a place with an atmosphere that's agreeable to you. At a friend's, you're greeted by the aromas of freshly prepared food coming from the kitchen. Perhaps you take a break from work at your favorite local café to enjoy the brew that the barista makes for you personally. Or soft candlelight makes you aware of a wooden dining table's lovely patina, peeking out from pleasing placemats.

Whether they're appealing or appalling, both the psycholog–ical mood and the physical accessories that surround you when you eat may influence the way in which you metabolize food—and, in turn, your health and well–being. Both are *externally* based, and both somehow impact your psyche and the way you metabolize your meals.

You may be surprised to learn that the atmosphere in which you eat can make a difference in your weight. In fact, implementing the antidotes to this eating style may quickly improve the quality of your life by enhancing how you feel both physically and emotionally. It may even improve your relationships—with others as well as with food. You'll focus on the psychological and physical aesthetics of your food life; the atmosphere in your home, in restaurants, and at drive–through restaurants; and the *quality* of companionship when you dine with family, friends, and coworkers—or by yourself. When you eat alone, are you taking the time to set a sumptuous table, play enjoyable music, and eat with a meditative mindset? Or are you eating pizza out of the cardboard box with the TV blasting in the background, dis–tracted by the details of daily life? In other words, are you providing nice company for yourself?

Enchanting Ingredients

Long before our research revealed the psychological and aesthetic ingredients of the unpleasant atmosphere eating style as a risk factor for weight gain, we had clues that atmosphere somehow makes a difference to our psyche—and, in turn, our health and well−being. One of the more memorable and exceptional dining environments we've experienced, one that brought a glow to heart and soul (and palate), awaited us in a private dining room at Statholdergaarden in Oslo, Norway, the restaurant of award−winning chef Bent Stiansen.

When we entered with our Norwegian friends Erik and Tine, we were greeted by an elegant, Continental atmosphere replete with chandeliers, candlelit tables, Oriental rugs covering polished wooden floors, portraits and landscape paintings on the walls, and the quiet conversation of elegantly garbed diners seated at antique wooden tables in various cozy dining rooms. Just as delightful were the menu lying like a crisp fall leaf at each place setting and the solicitous, gra−cious waiters who presented the vegetarian meal to us. Over the next five hours (yes, the meal lasted for five hours), course after course was served caringly and attentively. This was far more than a meal, we realized; it was an extraordinary dining event. Throughout the enchanted evening, waiters glided in and out unobtrusively, joining our conversation only to tell us about each course.

It's been more than ten years since that memorable meal in Norway, and we've eaten at many exceptional restaurants since then. Even so, that evening at Statholdergaarden, surrounded by excep−tional service, food, and friendship, still stands out as fare for heart and soul. And without a doubt, the enchanting psychological and aes−thetic environs had a lot to do with the evening's total nourishment.

While our culinary experience in Norway was exceptional, we've had comparable experiences during everyday meals with friends at their homes, in serendipitously discovered hole−in−the−wall restau−rants that served sublime food, and at meals in our own home. The homemade meals prepared by our friends David Leivick and Linda Gibbs in their seaside home in Northern California, for instance, always sparkle with freshness, flavor, and David's creativity and love of cooking. The food at the local Thai restaurant we stumbled onto one rainy

Sunday afternoon was so delicious and authentic that we felt we were in Thailand. Equally memorable are potluck Thanksgiving meals in our home that have been the culmination of friends' specialties; Peter's ten−ingredient salads are meals in themselves, Penny's cranberry sauce is a holiday luxury, and Vinita makes really mean desserts.

In contrast to such psychologically and aesthetically satisfying experiences, Americans currently eat about 20 percent of their meals inside their cars—often between errands or meetings. To accommo−date this growing group, the fast−food outlet In−N−Out Burger has developed paper "laptops" so that we can keep our clothes clean while we drive and eat. Whether we're enveloped in car fumes, fluorescent lighting, or abrasive noise, dining frequently in an unpleasant atmo−sphere contributes to a negative relationship with food and increased odds of growing girth.

The dining experience we had in Norway tells us that while food technology and what, how, and where we eat may have changed over the years, the kinds of surroundings that nourish our soul have not. What happens when the atmosphere in which we eat is jarring to the psyche? When both the psychological and the aesthetic surround−ings aren't just unwelcoming and unpleasant, but overtly hostile? An unusual study done just after World War II offers insight.

Hostile Ingredients

On June 16, 1951, the prestigious medical journal *The Lancet* pub−lished a study that couldn't be done today. Not only were children involved, but the conditions were so health−threatening—both emotionally and physically—that a modern−day review board would never approve the study design. In 1948 British nutritionist Elsie M. Widdowson was working at orphanages in Germany, where thou−sands of children had lost their families in World War II. It was a time of extreme trauma for the orphans, and their suffering was exacer−bated by food shortages and rationing.

While working at two orphanages, Widdowson was able to observe and record an extraordinary situation that evolved. Her one−year study started when she decided to monitor and measure the impact of addi−tional servings of food on the children's weight and height. Would those who received extra food gain more weight than those who received rations only? Would they grow taller than children who ate less? To find out, during the first six months Widdowson gave children at both orphanages equal food portions; during the second six–month period she fed children at one orphanage larger portions of bread, jam, and orange juice. Throughout the twelve months of the study, she weighed and measured the height of the children every ten days.

When she looked at the height and weight charts, Widdowson was perplexed. During the first six months, when everyone received equal portions, children at one orphanage had gained a lot more weight and had grown much more than children at the other orphanage. Things became even more confounding during the second six–month period, when the children who had been fed *more* food gained *less* weight and height than the others.

Widdowson pondered whether it was possible for children to thrive—or not—regardless of the quantity of food they ate. But when she scrutinized the atmosphere in both orphanages, she got an unexpected explanation for the seemingly contradictory results: Frau Schwarz. The children who'd failed to gain weight and grow had been overseen by a strict disciplinarian who chose mealtime to publicly ridicule and rebuke some of them. This explained the difference. "By the time she had finished," wrote Widdowson, "all the children would be in a state of considerable agitation, and several of them might be in tears."

Have you ever felt hungry, then lost your appetite because you were upset? Or did your food sit like a lump because you'd eaten while agitated? Perhaps you've eaten to stuff down feelings. The idea that your psychological state can influence digestion is now so familiar that it's easy to lose sight of how amazing Widdowson's findings were considered. But amazing they are. The discovery that children's psychological surroundings when they eat can determine whether they grow is remarkable—and It leads to the question of how a stress–filled environment influences the way we metabolize food and, in turn, our health. Answering this question calls for a rudimentary understanding of the process of digestion and the role that atmosphere and emotions can play.[1]

The Link between Stress and Poor Digestion

One of the most remarkable stories of how emotions can affect digestion starts in 1822, on Mackinac Island in Michigan, when an army surgeon named William Beaumont treated eighteen–year–old French Canadian fur trapper Alexis St. Martin for an accidental gun–shot wound to his stomach. Shot at close range, St. Martin was so seriously injured that Beaumont didn't expect him to survive. But not only did St. Martin live, but the major wound healed, except for a small opening in his stomach.

At the time, little was known about the process of digestion; it was a mystery discussed in the medical community in Europe, especially France. Ignorant of the debate that raged but intrigued by the puzzle of digestion, Beaumont turned St. Martin's mishap into ground–breaking observational studies: over a period of ten years, during which time he performed about 200 experiments, he became the first medical scientist to observe and carefully record a human being's digestive process.

What exactly occurred when food was digested? What were the elements of stomach acid? Beaumont documented it all. He was the first to show that digestion actually slowed down when someone was upset. How did this come about? Because Beaumont's observational studies were time–consuming and difficult—unpleasant and difficult to endure—St. Martin would become irritated. For instance, the only way Beaumont could observe digestion was to place food via a silk string into the opening in St. Martin's stomach and then remove it to observe any changes. And it was during one of these experiments that Beaumont observed that the food wasn't digested as well when St. Martin was upset.[2]

Since Beaumont's pioneering observations, science has made great strides in decoding the emotions/digestion puzzle—what behavioral scientists today might describe as the mind–body con–nection. Consider what happens when you eat while stressed, which was what happened to the children in Widdowson's experiment who failed to prosper. It will be helpful for you to know that while there are many definitions of "stress," we're defining it here as a "perceived threat" to either physical or emotional well–being.

Why does it matter if you eat while stressed out, when you're experiencing unpleasant emotions? When you do so, your brain releases a torrent of sometimes–contradictory hormones (chemical messengers) that put your digestive system in disarray. For instance, to give you strength for "fight or flight" in response to a perceived threat, you may manufacture the fat–friendly hormone *cortisol* or CRH (*corticotrophin*–releasing hormone), which in turn produces energy–giving adrenaline. CRH can also suppress your appetite (what seems to have happened to Widdowson's upset orphans), or it may have the opposite impact: it may produce steroids (organic fat–soluble compounds) that can make you hungry—and prompt you to overeat calorie–dense foods such as cookies, cake, or potato chips. In other words, an unpleasant psychological atmosphere can cause your body to produce hormones that prompt you to eat more.

Mealtime Emotions

Why have we been created with an amazingly strong connection between the brain and the digestive system—a relationship so pow–erful that the stomach and intestines are abundant in nerve cells, even more so than the spinal cord? Why has our mind–body been designed to pay such close attention to our environment and our emotions, with the ability to respond accordingly? Researcher Candace B. Pert explored the physical, emotional, and spiritual reasons for feelings.

Pert's pioneering work presents a scientific picture about how environment may influence digestion and increase the drive to overeat: in other words: stress more, eat more. The story starts with substances called *peptides*, which reside not only in the brain but throughout your entire body. And it is *neuropeptides* specifically that act as the biological foundation of the awareness we bring to meals— indeed, to all aspects of our lives.

What's unique about neuropeptides is that they are released into the bloodstream by *nerve cells*. The link to nerve cells is fascinating, because the hormones and other chemicals made by our mind–body create a two–way freeway that serves as a dynamic information net–work between the brain and the digestive system. Neuropeptides influence your experience of your world; and vice versa, your con–

sciousness—or mind, or emotions—affects your biology. Put another way, your body is strongly influenced by your emotions. Because of this, "the environment in which you eat has a lot to do with your emotional experience at mealtime," writes Pert. Eat in an unappe-tizing atmosphere, and "it's a kind of disintegration, *a mind-body split that will lead to weight gain* [italics ours] and disease conditions caused . . . by incomplete digestion."[3]

But there's another reason you're likely to eat more and gain weight when you consume food in an unpleasant psychological atmosphere: it influences the type (worse) and quantity (more) of food you eat. Researchers discovered this when they asked thirty subjects to watch *Love Story*, a sad movie that leads people to cry easily and often. As the study subjects watched the film, they ate 28 percent more buttered, salty popcorn (124.97 grams versus 97.97 grams) than they did while watching *Sweet Home Alabama*, a breezy comedy.[4] The same researchers found similar results with college stu-dents asked to read about children who died in a fire. As they read the heartbreaking news, they ate four times more M&M's than raisins from nearby bowls of snacks. In contrast, when the same students read about a delightful chance reunion among four old friends, they *didn't* turn to unhealthful food, but rather to healthful snacks. The message: if you want to eat less and weigh less, refrain from using the dinner table as a place to argue or scold or to think about unpleasant things.

Food and Fuel

Plenty of situations lend themselves to creating an aesthetically unpleasant and discordant eating atmosphere. Consider this common scenario. You're driving in Anywhere, USA, and pull into a gas station. When you get out of your car to fuel up, a sign tells you that you need to pay inside. As you walk past other motorists filling their tanks, you cringe slightly as you register the potent smell of petroleum.

Feeling a bit queasy from the odor, you walk inside to prepay. Your nostrils are instantly filled with the scent of rancid cooking oil; at the same time, the harshness of the overhead fluorescent lighting causes you to squint a bit. While waiting in line, you glance at the TV on the counter that's blasting bad news. You're also privy to a distasteful discussion between the cashier and the customer in front of you, who claims he's been shortchanged. You look around to locate the source of the unappetizing aroma and realize it's coming from a fast–food outlet that shares space with the gasoline station store. You notice a customer eating a hamburger and fries as he walks out the door toward his car. He'll probably eat while driving, you think as you continue to wait.

Such "cobranded on–site locations"—the merger of fast food and a gas station, or two or more fast–food restaurants under one roof—are common sights and eating experiences for many Americans. Think about the last gas station store you entered that was abundant with packaged junk food, the last fast–food restaurant where you ate, or the last convenience store you went to for a late–night snack. Were you aware of the subtle assault the atmosphere was making on your psyche and the way it was impacting your digestive system, your entire being?

Optimal Healing Environments

Although it's still an emerging field, the medical community is becoming more and more aware that environment has a pro–found impact on health and healing. The movement is gaining such momentum that at the second Symposium on Optimal Healing Environments sponsored by the Samueli Institute, physician and author Larry Dossey described the study of healing environments as a "huge social movement whose momentum is unstoppable." More than fifty scientists and clinicians were invited to the event to define "healing environments" and challenges related to creating them.

Intrigued, we studied the symposium topics, which addressed environments for disciplines as diverse as nursing, integrative medi–cine, and health care in general, as well as for ailments ranging from chronic cardiovascular disease and chronic low–back pain to cancer and childhood obesity. Given our own research and the unappetizing atmosphere eating style we'd identified, the presentation that really caught our attention was the work of Marc Schweitzer and colleagues, because it identified specific environmental elements that make an impact on health. "The 'ambiance' of a space has an effect on people

146

using the space," Schweitzer states. And then he identifies elements that are integral to a healing environment: personal space; sound/noise; temperature; fresh air and ventilation; enjoyable social interaction (social support); warm, natural light; color; a view and experience of nature; arts, aesthetics, and entertainment (such as music).[5]

We were especially interested in Schweitzer's overview of the elements of a healing environment, because throughout this chapter we're suggesting that the atmosphere in which you eat can be either healing (by increasing the odds of optimal digestion and, in turn, optimal weight and well-being) or harmful (by increasing the odds of poor digestion or overeating, thus contributing to weight gain). Throughout the day you have plenty of nonhealing opportunities to assault your psyche and system (and waistline) by eating in an abrasive atmosphere. The gas station situation described above was replete with harsh lighting, contrary people, and depressing news blaring from the TV. Add cramped quarters, stuffy and stale air, and a motley collection of disparate food products and car accoutrements, and you have the antithesis of the healing environment that Schweitzer described.

Optimal Eating Atmosphere

Most of us know that eating in congenial surroundings is, at the very least, enjoyable. This is good news, since you can access or create delightful surroundings anytime. Envision a fall picnic, for instance, surrounded by the colors of the season in the leaves and in the deep orange of pumpkin soup. Or think of the soothing comfort of a homemade stew eaten in winter as candlelight flickers and you're surrounded by steamed-up windows, while outside a blanket of snow covers your yard. Imagine an impromptu meal of pasta, salad, and wine made with friends when a sudden spring shower abates. Or picture a summer salad sprinkled with edible and organic flowers.

The possibilities are endless. Yet the role that ambiance and your surroundings play in overeating and indigestion problems continues to be an overlooked aspect of well-being. What would an optimal psychological and aesthetic eating environment look like? Here are some suggestions for creating an affable dining milieu, as often as possible.

Limit lighting. One of our favorite restaurants has low–hanging lights above each booth, which we find harsh. Each time we eat there, we think about how much more we'd enjoy the meal and the entire dining experience if, instead, it were infused with candlelight. When you eat at home, diffuse the light by turning on a nearby lamp, dim–ming your overhead light, or eating by candlelight.

Walk away. A friend of mine told me that not too long after she read our research paper on the overeating styles[6], she was feeling hypo–glycemic (weak from low blood sugar) and hungry in the middle of the day while "choring." She made the spontaneous decision to buy a sweet from a gourmet cookie shop to quickly appease her hunger. But she was dissuaded from staying by the acid rock music that blasted from speakers and the uninterested clerks who talked among them–selves instead of taking her order. She found a friendlier place down the block for a midday munch. When you eat out—whether it's a full meal or a munchie—choose an amiable place whenever possible.

Cherish china. When Oprah did a show on "anti–aging break–throughs," a weight–loss lifestyle was one of the topics. To high–light the elements of her successful weight loss, an audience member shared her personal success story. Along with moving more and choosing fresh food, the aesthetic atmosphere she created was part of her twenty–two–pound weight loss. I put my portion [of food] on beautiful plates, with great style, lovely linens, crystal, [and] china, and enjoyed every morsel," she said. "No more standing in the kitchen eating out of a little container."[7] Whenever possible, eat on quality plates with your best utensils, and sit down at a dining table to enjoy your meal even more.

Rest, relax. A friend of ours who is a *yogini* (a woman who practices yoga) told us that after she shared a large lunch in the home of a revered family in India, her hosts invited her to lie down and rest so that she could digest the meal in a peaceful and quiet environment. In a time– and work–driven country such as ours, this isn't a realistic option, but what we can do is a modified version: after eating, take the time to enjoy some easygoing conversation with others, relaxing music, or an enjoyable article.

Release emotions. Thanks to Candace Pert's research on emo‒tions and digestion, it's safe to say that the psychological atmosphere in which you eat influences the way you metabolize food and, in turn, your weight and well‒being. That's why you'll find it helpful to release toxic molecules of emotion when you eat. If you find yourself ruminating about something unpleasant, put your emotions on hold and press the pause button as you eat; instead, think about some‒thing agreeable. You can always return to the problem later. Or, if the people with whom you're dining are more negative than positive, try to redirect the conversation by asking them to share something that's working well or is enjoyable in their lives.

Eat outside. If you have access to a park near your house, outdoor dining tables and chairs in the courtyard where you work, or a café that enables you to eat outdoors, take advantage of the opportu‒nity to enjoy fresh air and beautiful surroundings. And there's another benefit: you can get a little exercise while walking to your favorite outdoor eating place. (See Chapter 11, "Get Moving," for more ideas about including more movement in your life.)

Dine by Design
The psychological and aesthetic environments connected to food and eating may be the most over‒looked aspect of weight gain, but as we've seen throughout this chapter, it is a powerful determinant of your weight. Commit to taking charge by "designing" the most pleasant ambiance possible each time you eat.

Unappetizing atmosphere Rx: Dine in psychologically and aesthetically pleasing surroundings.

We weren't surprised when our research showed unappetizing atmo‒sphere to be linked with overeating. What astonished us was that, as with all the overeating styles, it was statistically significant: it's not due to chance that when you eat in an unappetizing atmosphere, you're at increased risk for weight gain. To achieve and maintain optimal weight, we've given you lots of guidelines for dining in psycho-logically and aesthetically pleasing surroundings that are inherently healing and healthy.

Chapter 8

Feed the Senses

We experienced the power of feeding the senses, especially taste, long before we identified sensory disregard as one of the overeating styles. It was while we were having dinner in a beautiful Thai restaurant, where we'd ordered a salad with which we weren't familiar. Called *miang kam*, the dish that arrived at our table wasn't the familiar American salad of mixed vegetables. Instead, we were presented with a platter that held six small bowls filled with finely chopped and colorful ingredients: lime, peanuts, red onion, red pepper, ginger, and toasted coconut. In the center were a bunch of fresh spinach leaves and a bowl of a very thick and sticky sweet–and–sour paste.

The presentation was enchanting, but because it was also unfamiliar, we asked our waitress how we should proceed. Patiently she showed us how to take a spinach leaf, spread a little paste on it, and sprinkle a tiny portion from each bowl over the paste. Then she created a small food–filled tube by rolling up the leaf. When we tasted the handmade tubular salad, our taste buds burst with flavor. With each bite, an implosion of flavors was released, so much so that we kept our attention and our anticipation focused on the fantastic flavors and tantalizing tastes that each new *miang kam* released.

Our *miang kam* dining experience is an exceptional example of how fresh food, prepared with care and savored by the diner, can fill the senses and satisfy the soul—the two key ingredients lacking in the sensory disregard eating style. We're especially excited to tell you about this eating style because our research is the first to reveal the sensory and spiritual elements—which go together like twins—of eating and overeating.

When you take time to experience your food through all your senses—taste (flavor), smell (aroma), sight (presentation), sound (of the surroundings), and touch (*kinesthetics*)—and to regard the mystery of life inherent in food and in yourself, you're more likely to be truly nourished and less likely to overeat. Dining with your senses (sensory *regard*) and at the same time eating with a deep appreciation for the food before you (spiritual *connection*) are powerful ways to nurture and nourish yourself—and, in turn, to feel fulfilled by the dining experience. When you do this, you're likely to eat less and enjoy it more.

Sensory Disregard, Spiritual Disconnection

Regard for and connection to eating are the antithesis of how many who struggle with weight relate to food. What's more typical is sensory *dis*regard and spiritual *dis*connection. What does this eating style look like? If you've ever eaten quickly and mindlessly and scarfed down food—perhaps you've let yourself become super hungry, or depressed emotions are dictating what and how you eat—then you've eaten without experiencing the color, aroma, flavor, texture, presentation, and portion size of your food. This is sensory disregard. And if you typically eat without reflecting on the mystery of food's ability to sustain life; if you ignore the way rain, sunshine, wind, and soil work together to create the foods that nourish you; and if you don't stop to appreciate, from the heart, the origins of the food before you—then you are eating with spiritual disconnection.

The idea that eating with sensory disregard and spiritual disconnection can lead to weight gain may seem somewhat unusual. After all, the seemingly simple calories in/calories out formula discussed in Chapter 2, "Jettison Judgment," is the standard solution to weight loss that most health professionals offer: just cut down on the amount of food you eat and move more, and you'll lose weight. Eating with your senses and connecting to the meaning in meals, on the other hand, isn't so straightforward. Rather, it requires you to replace caloriecounting with sensory and sensual pleasure, and to transform phobic food thoughts ("I can't eat that; it's fattening") into a world filled with the wonder and delight of eating, and into a relationship with food that includes appreciating the meaning and mystery of life inherent in your meals.

Surely most of us don't flavor our meals with sensory and spiritual delight. And we're paying a big price with our growing girth. While vacationing in Mexico, *San Francisco Chronicle* columnist Mark Morford observed many overweight Americans. He considered the sensory and spiritual starvation that is normal for many Americans, and its link with being overweight, and he speculated about the detachment so many overweight people must feel from their bodies—a spiritual emptiness and lack of true nourishment—even as they're overeating.[1]

You can fill a sense of spiritual vacuity, a lack of true nourish-ment, if you take the time to taste your food and to appreciate the multidimensional ways it nourishes you. Each time you eat, savor the flavors in your food.

Sacred Scents

A time-tested example of the way humankind has always turned to the senses to satisfy the soul is Judaism's sacred scents ceremony. Toward dusk on Saturday, after a day of resting, thinking, reading, or playing (just *being* rather than *doing*), the Jewish Sabbath ends when three stars can be seen in the sky. This transition—between the Sabbath and the other days of the week—is celebrated with blessings. Called *havdalah*, meaning "separation," the informal farewell calls for a cup filled with wine, a candle, and a box of spices (*besamin*).

"May the coming week overflow with goodness like the wine in the cup," says the head of the household, holding the *kiddish* cup as it brims with wine. Then comes the lighting of a special candle, made of twisted strands symbolizing the many different kinds of light God has created (the sun, moon, and stars, and the Jewish laws by which to live). Next, a spice box (a replacement for the incense-burning of ancient times) is opened, releasing the fragrant scent of cloves, nutmeg, and bay leaves—symbolizing hope for a week that will be pleasant and sweet smelling.

Judaism's brief *havdalah* ceremony signifying the end of Shabbat is rich in the inhalation of sweet and savory spices. Its purpose is to capture the senses and serve as a reminder to hold onto moments of sweetness and peace during the busy work week. Such symbolism has its roots in the *neshama yeterah*—the second, extra soul Jews are believed to acquire during Shabbat—which enhances the ability to rejoice in tranquility and to live with a feeling of contentment. The holiness and intention of the day is one of *oneg Shabbat*—the joy, pleasure, relaxation, and ease of the Sabbath.

When Shabbat draws to a close, tradition holds that the extra soul withdraws, leaving the mundane soul in its place. Because it's believed that aromas from the material world are the only aspect that the everyday, remaining soul can enjoy, the spice box and its scents serve to console and connect with the remaining soul throughout the week. In this way, inhaling the sacred aromatics signifies more than the moment of transition from the spiritual to the material world: it also fills our being with the spicy sweetness of each moment. As these sacred scents capture the senses and provide a mindful pause, we are empowered to hold on to the peaceful, meaningful memory of the Sabbath—until next Friday at sunset.

Flavor-Full Weight Loss

Perhaps Judaism's havdalah ceremony evolved with the intuitive understanding that slowing down and taking the time to savor scents is one path to spiritual satisfaction. But might it lead to weight loss, as our study on the seven overeating styles suggests? Perhaps the best example of the way in which "eating with your senses" may lead to weight loss is evident in the work of psychologist Seth Roberts, emeritus professor of psychology at the University of California at Berkeley. While reviewing scientific journals in preparation for a lecture, Roberts had an "Aha!" insight. Might it be possible, he wondered, that the amount of body fat you have is linked to—even controlled by—the flavor in the food you eat? Somehow, might the brain depend on the flavor in food to gauge how much fat your body stores (leading to weight gain) or releases (leading to weight loss)?[2]

At the time, Roberts's reasoning was derived from insights into human beings' evolution as well as state-of-the-art brain research.[3] Isn't it likely, he thought, that when we eat a lot of tasty, tempting, high−calorie food (such as ice cream, donuts, or potato chips), our brain thinks this is a time of abundance (translation: a caveman has just killed a tiger, and food will be plentiful for a while)? Then, to ensure we'll survive during times of scarcity, our brain tells our body to stockpile the pounds you put on from the food.

In essence, Roberts is saying that flavorful food triggers "an increase in hunger and fat storage. By contrast, not−so−mouthwa− tering or flavorless calories signal scarcity." He is suggesting that when you consume simple, unflavored food (he uses cooking oil, such as canola, as an example, but iceberg lettuce, steamed rice, or air− popped popcorn also illustrate the idea), your brain gets the message that you're not too hungry and therefore you eat less, making it easy for stored fat to be released.[4]

To put his interesting idea into action, Roberts used his own mind−body . . . and taste buds. Our friend and colleague Keri Brenner, a journalist and author specializing in health and Complementary and Alternative Medicine (CAM), interviewed Roberts for an article about his Shangri−La Diet. Brenner was interested in writing about Roberts's work because he claimed he had lost fifty pounds by having either a tablespoon of oil or a cup of water sweetened with a table− spoon of sugar (fructose) between meals. He told Brenner he'd actu− ally had to gain back ten pounds, because over a long period of time he'd become too thin. Now, to maintain his weight loss, he eats one meal a day, with small snacks such as fruit during the day and still taking the oil or sugar water—but not as frequently—and he claims he isn't hungry for more than that.

Does Roberts' flavor−based theory hold up? Intrigued by a newspaper article she'd read about the plan, Brenner decided to find out. "I thought it was unusual and interesting, because it's not a tra− ditional diet," she told us, "and it doesn't involve any special menus or calorie−counting; there's no exercise, or any of the other usual weight−loss 'suspects.'" She was also interested in the Shangri−La Diet for personal reasons. "I've always struggled with the usual extra five or ten pounds," she said, citing a common problem for women. Brenner has dabbled with different diets and exercise regimens over the years. Could the "no hunger, eat anything plan" espoused by Roberts really make a difference? Here's Brenner's experience:

> I gave up baked goods and bread seven years ago, because I have a predisposition to overeat refined carbs and sugars and then gain weight. And I don't feel good. Roberts' plan was appealing because it sounded simple and easy. All I had to do to follow his program was to take measured doses of dull, unflavored food, such as one cup of fructose—flavored water or one tablespoon of fla—vorless extra—light olive oil, in between meals, two to four times a day; you can do either one. As part of the plan, I also couldn't eat or drink or even brush my teeth with peppermint toothpaste for an hour before or after taking the oil or sugar—water, so that I wouldn't contaminate my palate with other tastes.
>
> During the first week after I started the diet, I was in a restau—rant with my husband, and the grilled fish and salad combination arrived. I took a bite, and I knew I was actually meditating. It was that intense. My whole mouth was filled with the flavor of the food, and the experience of eating was much richer, more intense, and satisfying than usual. I was almost experiencing the chef pre—paring the food, all the care that went into creating these fla—vors; I had an appreciation of the food in every way. I remember thinking that somebody really put a lot of regard and care into the food. When I took a bite, I was instantly connected to the whole creation of the food; much more so than normal. And I think I experienced this because it was such a strong contrast to the fla—vorless food. It was transcendent; truly.
>
> Did the plan take away my hunger? Absolutely, it did—[espe—cially] for mindless snacking. But I would be hungry for healthy food—salads, proteins, and other fresh foods. Then, when I would eat a meal, I had a much greater appreciation for the flavors in the food. When I ate, I seemed to experience more pleasure and awareness. I would take a bite, and the flavor would be inten—sified. As a consequence, I ate less because I felt more satisfied when I ate, because I appreciated the flavors in the food. I also ate more fresh food. For me, Roberts' theory works. I lost four or

five pounds during the first month, without trying. I also lost my appetite for random snacking and grazing on nuts, trail mix, and protein bars while at work. On the other hand, I gained a greater appreciation of fresh food, and how it tasted. I stopped eating on autopilot and started to look forward to deliberately paying attention to what I was eating, and to the flavors. I wasn't trying to do this; it just happened.

Brenner told us she followed the plan for about three months but tapered off after a while, because her schedule got too hectic. She just didn't have the time to continue taking the oil and sugar–water supplements. Soon she got out of the habit of supplementing with oil or sugar water during the day. And when she returned to her regular way of eating, not surprisingly the weight returned. Still, Brenner thinks that if you can stick to the regimen, at the least your ability to enjoy healthy foods and their natural flavors will increase. "I don't know if the Shangri–La Diet is the answer to all the factors that con– tribute to overeating and weight gain," she reflected, "but I do know that when I followed the technique, I lost weight."[5]

What does focusing on flavors in food suggest about food, eating, and your weight? It tells us that food, in part, is a function of its fla– vors, and that when you take the time to savor flavors and truly taste all elements of your meal, an invisible but soul–satisfying dynamic somehow nourishes you. You don't have to solve all aspects of your relationship to food to achieve and maintain a normal weight: you can lower the odds of overeating and weight gain just by focusing on the flavors in your food.

Roberts' "flavor theory" also confirms the problems inherent in the food fretting eating style of traditional dieting based on a pre– scribed food regimen. Even if Roberts isn't suggesting a traditional diet, what he's proposing is still, well, a diet. And as Brenner experi– enced when she went off the oil or sugar–water regimen, her former eating habits and weight returned.

If we take a closer look at the "transcendent" eating experi– ence she had while focusing on flavors, we can get a better sense of the "spiritual disconnection" half of this eating style, and how you can use it to your advantage to overcome overeating. By listening to this invisible mind—body message, you're likely to replace eating on autopilot with the amount of food your body really needs. Isn't it amazing? Simply by focusing on the flavors in your food, you may be less likely to overeat and gain weight.

Meals of Mystery and Meaning

We vividly remember the moment we were introduced to the idea that a spiritual, meaningful connection to food has been integral to humankind for millennia. We were in New Delhi, India, where we had been invited to give a workshop at the First International Conference on Lifestyle and Health. During a discussion with Hindu cardiologist Dr. K. L. Chopra, father and mentor of the well—known author Deepak Chopra, he told us that the *Bhagavad Gita*, Hindu scripture, presents *prana*, the vital life force of the universe, as a cosmic consciousness that is metabolized when we eat. When you cook, you transfer your emo—tions into the food; in turn, when you eat the food, you metabolize the consciousness, or *prana*, with which the food was prepared.

Fascinated by the possibility that consciousness could alter the food we eat, we began a search to unearth wisdom about the pro—found meaning of food in our lives—to examine food and eating in the light of spiritual sustenance, to explore the interconnectedness between human consciousness and food. What we discovered is that in most world views, food has been surrounded with sacred sym—bolism and spiritual beliefs for centuries.

Food was considered hallowed by the early Israelites, a means to worship Allah by the Muslims, and a medium for transmitting psychic substance between individuals by the Hindus. In the Christian com—munity, the Eucharist (from the Greek *eucharisto*, "to give thanks") uses bread and wine to connect to deeper mysteries. "We cannot see the secret vital force . . . which gives life to the grape and the grain," wrote mystic and nun Hildegard of Bingen in the twelfth century. "Yet the same force is at work when the bread and wine of the Eucharist are transformed into the flesh and blood of Christ."[6]

Though it is usually only a bite of bread and a swallow of wine (or juice) that contemporary Christians consume when they receive the Eucharist (or take Communion), the meal is rich in many ways. Multidimensional nourishment is present when participants are fed physically with bread and beverage, nourished emotionally by being part of something holy, filled spiritually by experiencing Jesus' god—liness, and satisfied socially through sharing sustenance with others. (For more about the four facets of food that nourish body, mind, soul, and social well—being, see the book Introduction, "Make Weight Loss Last: The 10 Solutions.")

The belief that a divine power could be ingested has its roots with early pagans, who practiced a ritual of sacrifice wherein they actu—ally ingested parts of the body of an animal that represented a certain god. When Jesus took bread and wine, blessed it, and said, "This is my body" and "This is my blood . . . which is to be poured out for many," he was walking the well—trodden path of those pre—Christian sacrificial rites. He was pursuing and obtaining spiritual sustenance through a profoundly meaningful, super—conscious awareness of, and connection to, the mystery of life inherent in humans and in the nourishment that is food.

Filling the Void

When we discussed Barbara Birsinger's research on emotional eating in Chapter 4, "Access Your Appetite," we talked about the differ—ence between a nutritional craving (for protein or carbohydrates, for example) and a craving based on uncomfortable emotions (such as loneliness, anger, or anxiety). With the sensory disregard overeating style, we aren't addressing emotions; we're alluding to a deep, internal hunger for something more intangible than food. Often that "some—thing more" translates into profound yearning for spiritual sustenance; a longing to fill that empty feeling and lack of meaning and purpose in our lives; and a need to have a deeper connection with ourselves and others—indeed, the world.

Aware of the spiritual element of overeating, Birsinger invited the Reverend Josephine Smith to work with participants in her study by helping them feel more spiritually fulfilled through meditation, prayer, and spiritual community. If someone in the group needed to talk during the session, Smith was available to work with that person one on one.

Spiritual connection is so integral to Birsinger's program that she called it "Conversations with Bod: Discovering the Spiritual Archetypal and Symbolic Messages in Food, Eating, Body Language, and Weight." Her rationale: longtime food restrictors, or those who live on a restriction–bingeing cycle, need to get in touch with their own biology again. "There's a disconnection from the body," Birsinger says, "a disconnect at the neck. The more severe the eating disorder, the more severe is the disconnection. Once a person gets to this point, a structured, regular eating plan is needed so the body can be reminded again about what it feels like to be hungry or full. Once they can feel and sense their internal hunger and satiety signals, they're able to learn and implement Intuitive Eating and get well."[7]

Birsinger helps people fill a spiritual void by showing them how to "shift focus from the external world around eating to an internal one," in other words by becoming aware of why we make the food choices we do. The next step is to learn that the food choices we make have an important purpose; this gives people a sense of accep-tance and compassion for themselves regarding their eating habits and behaviors. The big shift, she says, "is realizing how food has been serving as a way to take care of yourself. Once people get this, it's an epiphany; they realize that can change. And when this happens, it leads to optimal eating and weight loss."[8]

Sensory Regard Strategies

We've already discussed what it means to "eat with your senses" by taking in the colors, textures, and aromas of food, for example. But did you know that Eastern healing systems such as India's Ayurveda, tra-ditional Chinese medicine (TCM), and Tibetan Medicine have turned to six flavors in food to signal optimal eating and complete nutrition?

We had been familiar with the role of the six tastes in Ayurveda and TCM, but we discovered their place in Tibetan Medicine during a lecture by Tibetan physician Dr. Namgyal Qusar. In response to a question from the audience about optimal food preparation and nutrient preservation, Dr. Qusar responded by clarifying the Tibetan concept of "balance," consuming food from all food groups—both plant— and animal—based. Then he added that for complete nutrition, you have to eat all six tastes: sweet, sour, salty, bitter, pungent, and astrin— gent. In other words, Tibetan nutrition uses a finely honed sense of taste to ascertain whether a meal is balanced—and to find out, you have to focus your attention on the flavors inside your mouth as you chew.[9]

The six tastes are so integral to health and well—being in Ayurveda that some ancient Ayurvedic schools encourage a sequence of tastes in a meal, progressing from sweet to salty, sour, pungent, bitter, and then astringent.

Savor six tastes. To put the concept of the six tastes into practice, gather the ingredients to make the unique Thai appetizer salad called *miang kam* (described earlier in this chapter): one each **lime**, small **red onion**, and **red bell pepper**; a piece of **ginger**; two tablespoons shredded and toasted **coconut**; some **honey** (perhaps 1/4 cup); and about ten **spinach leaves**.

Chop the lime, onion, pepper, and ginger into tiny pieces. Next, spread a thin layer of honey (perhaps a teaspoon) on one spinach leaf, then sprinkle a pinch of each chopped ingredient over the sticky honey. Roll up the spinach leaf, creating a small food—filled tube.

With your eyes closed, take a bite and begin to chew. Focus solely on the food in your mouth. Can you taste fantastic flavors? Are you able to identify one or more of the six tastes? Simply appreciate every single flavor.

Engage your senses. Experiencing food with your senses can con— nect you to the sacred, to the mystery of life, to other beings (indeed, to "being"). It's possible to nourish yourself this way with one of humankind's simplest and most basic foods, bread—whether you're eating a sandwich with friends, buttering bread at a restaurant, or having friends or family members over to create communion by sharing bread, cheese, and fruit in your home.

Making such a meaningful connection calls for engaging all your senses: sight, touch, smell, taste, and hearing. *Look* at the bread you're going to eat and become aware of its texture and color. Is it smooth, rough, light, dark? When you take the bread in your hands, what does it *feel* like? Is it soft, tough, grainy? Next identify the *smell* of the bread. Is it sweet? Sour? In between? When you take a bite, do you *taste* one or more flavors? (Hint: the taste of food often changes as you chew.) Finally, how does the bread you're chewing *sound*? Loud, or subtle?

Each time you break bread is an opportunity to be nourished spiritually. But the extent to which this connection is revealed to you depends on your heartfelt intention and the degree to which you are willing to infuse bread—and all food and eating—with the mystery of sensory regard.

Connection Strategies

The antidote to sensory disregard and spiritual disconnection lies in discovering how to "eat from a place of spirit." This phrase coined by clinical psychologist Michael Mayer means that when you eat, you access *chi*, a centuries–old concept from China that describes the life force within all living things, from feelings to food. When you cultivate *chi*, "you merge with the mysterious energy source in the world that is life itself," says Mayer. And because such a comprehen–sive connection soothes the soul, it holds the power to fill the sense of emptiness that drives many of us to overeat.[10]

Earlier we told you about Judaism's havdalah ceremony, which captures the senses as a reminder to hold on to the Sabbath's moments of sweetness and peace during the busy work week. Bringing sim–ilar regard to food and the entire experience of dining means you're eating from the heart. This might be described in Hebrew as *yetzirah*, the spiritual awareness of unity and connection. And it is this under–standing, recognition, and perception that will fill and nourish heart and soul.

Eat like a yogi. Devout yogis—people who practice yoga—follow a philosophy of *Sanatana dharma*, the Sanskrit expression for the underlying, eternal, true essence of all life. Such a philosophy com–plements the *Bhagavad Gita*, which encourages honoring all living things—including food—as part of an interdependent oneness. With such a focus, the consciousness you bring to food may be the most important ingredient in the meal. When preparing or cooking food, think positive, loving, appreciative thoughts. Such a mentality may be transferred into the food, enhance digestion, and empower the food to nourish body, mind, and soul.

Like vitamins and minerals in life—giving foods, negative thoughts are believed to be metabolized, too. Avoid eating when you're angry, because negative thoughts are believed to create toxins that eventually will be secreted by the glands. Also, anger or stress may limit the production of digestive enzymes in our stomachs, making it difficult for food to be adequately digested. (See Chapter 7, "Dine by Design," for more about this.)

Brahman is the Sanskrit word that attempts to describe the indescribable; "a supreme, blissful consciousness" only hints at its meaning. Such a noble frame of mind is believed to contribute to optimal digestion. Just before eating, meditate on the following verse from the *Bhagavad Gita* (4:24), which expresses *Brahman* this way:

> The process of eating is Brahman;
> The offering [of food] is Brahman.
> The person offering is Brahman,
> And the fire is also Brahman.
> Thus by seeing Brahman everywhere in action,
> He [alone] reaches Brahman.

Experience a Eucharist consciousness. Most religions and cultures have developed rituals that use food to connect to a deeper significance. Communion, believed to transform (literally or symbolically) bread and wine into Jesus' body and blood, provides an opportunity for Christian believers to experience a profound spiritual connection through food. In part, it includes connecting to the Divine through a ritual that engages all the senses: sight, hearing, touch, smell, and taste.

Spiritual connection may manifest in other ways. During the Thanksgiving holiday, millions of Americans gather together to share food and thanks with family and friends. As we consume the lavish meal of turkey and dressing, potatoes, cranberries, and pumpkin pie,

163

we are honoring and connecting with the harvest of 1621, when about fifty settlers at Plymouth Colony invited approximately a hundred neighboring Native Americans to celebrate a much-appreciated crop of corn, barley, and peas. These were friends who had helped them through hard times. Imagine the gratitude in their hearts during this meal!

Make each meal meaningful. As with our friend Keri Brenner's transcendent dining experience—or the aesthetics of tea mind, the scents of the Sabbath, living a Eucharist consciousness, or Larry's special birthday celebration at Statholdergaarden—it's possible to make each meal a feast for both the senses and the soul. Accomplishing this calls for "charging the *chi*" by approaching food from that "place of spirit." When you eat with such heartfelt regard, you open the door to feeling connected to yourself and others—to the entire universe. And as you become more and more connected to your true nature, you make it more and more possible for your natural, normal weight to manifest.

Grow your own food. Growing the food that you cook creates a strong connection with the land and the seasons. If you don't have space to garden, consider a windowsill herb garden. Or buy food from your local farmers' market to experience the sensual pleasures of fresh, seasonal food; at the same time, you'll get to meet and appreciate the people who grow or make the food.

Feed the Senses

With this discussion of sensory disregard in eating, we've addressed the final overeating style. Incorporating a spiritual ingredient to help make weight loss last calls for creating a meaningful connection to food by appreciating all that went into bringing it to you, and savoring the flavors of each meal you eat. Here's the antidote for the sensory disregard eating style:

Sensory Disregard Rx: "Feed" your senses when you eat by savoring flavors, aromas, colors, presentation, textures, even sounds.

Our research on the seven overeating styles highlights the mis-take many make in thinking about eating and weight loss, which is the belief that a simple formula—eat less, move more—will cure the problem. Such a conviction underestimates the complexity of people's food choices and eating behaviors. We overeat and are over-weight for many reasons, from food fretting, task snacking, and emo-tional eating to fast foodism, solo dining, unpleasant atmosphere, and spiritual disconnection. But armed with the step-by-step strategies we've outlined, you can overcome your own overeating style by cre-ating a whole person nutrition plan based on your personal needs and health goals.

Chapter 9

Quit Chemical Cuisine

Most of us are familiar with the usual suspects in America's obesity epidemic—bucket-sized servings of buttered movie-house popcorn, supersized fast-food meals, driving when we could walk. As genuine as these problems are, they don't account for the fattening up of a significant new segment of the population, one that can't even pick up and chew a candy bar: infants.

Though most six-month-olds have a diet that consists largely of formula or breast milk and they spend much waking time moving their newly familiar bodies, the prevalence of obesity in infants rose 73 percent between 1980 and 2006, say scientists at the Harvard School of Public Health.[1] If conventional explanations for America's growing girth don't apply to infants, what might explain the stunning increase in their rate of obesity?

Unraveling the Mystery

If we look closely at the alarming increase in overweight infants, young children, teens, and adults, we learn that one of the key contributors came to light unexpectedly from a seemingly simple study. The discovery of a potential new cause of obesity began in 1993 when endocrinologist Dr. David Feldman and his team at the Stanford University School of Medicine set out to study whether yeast could produce estrogen, a naturally occurring hormone that acts as a key chemical messenger throughout the body.

To test their yeast-estrogen theory, the researchers designed a relatively simple study: they would add water and nutrients to

Saccharomyces cerevisiae, the yeast commonly used to bake bread and brew beer. Would the yeast bind with estrogen receptors? If so, it could mean that yeast—one of the simplest and most commonplace organisms on earth—does, indeed, create estrogen.

To prepare for their experiment, Feldman and his team needed to ensure that the water they were using was free of any contaminants or live organisms. To accomplish this, they sterilized already–distilled water in a hard plastic flask made of polycarbonate, a tough and ver–satile plastic used for a multitude of items—from baby bottles, canned foods, and bottled water containers to compact discs (CDs), eyeglasses, and cell phone and laptop casings. Soon a mysterious finding emerged: when Feldman studied the properties of the yeast medium, he found an alien, estrogen–like molecule that couldn't have come from the yeast. What was it, and how had it worked its way into the study?

To trace the source of the strange molecule, Feldman used two highly sensitive instruments (nuclear magnetic resonance spectros–copy and mass spectrometry) capable of identifying any chemicals in the water he'd sterilized. The molecule he ultimately identified was bisphenol A (BPA), an insidious compound that is the building block of polycarbonate plastic. Apparently the bisphenol A had leached out of the plastic flask when Feldman heated the water to a high temperature.

A New Health–Harmer

If Feldman had stopped his study with the mere discovery that the strange compound he'd found was BPA, we might still be in the dark about the silent ways in which BPA can threaten health and weight. But because he knew that BPA appeared to act like estrogen, Feldman and his team decided to see if the concentration of BPA that had leached into highly heated water was capable of triggering a response in human cancer cells. If so, it might mean that BPA could contribute to the progression of cancer.

What he found was staggering in its implications: even at very low concentrations (10 to 25 billionths of a *mole*, a molecular weight in grams), BPA activated receptor sites of the hormone proges–terone, which in turn can increase production of breast cancer cells in humans. In other words, "because of its estrogenic hormonelike properties, BPA has the potential to be important and perhaps even dangerous to people who were eating or drinking out of containers made of this type of plastic, polycarbonate."[2]

Since Feldman's breakthrough finding, more than 100 independently funded studies have added evidence of BPA's harmful health effects. Even at low— and short—term doses, exposure to BPA has been linked with increased risk of an alarming number of developmental, neural, and reproductive ailments in infants, children, and adults. A sampling includes breast cancer, prostate disease and cancer, heart disease, stroke, diabetes, hyperactivity, miscarriage, lowered sperm count and sperm defects, and Down's syndrome. And increasingly, BPA is being linked with obesity as well.[3-9]

Health threats linked with exposure to BPA are so pervasive that years after Feldman's discovery, academic environmentalist Theo Colborn, co—author of the landmark book *Our Stolen Future*, stated that BPA is the pollutant about which she is most concerned.[10] Her concern likely stems from these three facts: (1) billions of pounds of BPA are produced annually, and the amount continues to increase; (2) it's in so many products that most of us are constantly exposed to it; and (3) it affects every physiological system that's been studied so far.

The evidence linking overweight, obesity, and a plethora of health problems with the ingestion of BPA is so strong that regulatory agencies in Canada have declared BPA "a toxic chemical requiring aggressive action to limit human and environmental exposures," says Frederick vom Saal of the Division of Biological Sciences at the University of Missouri at Columbia. Studies by vom Saal, the leading researcher on the impact of small concentrations of endocrine disrupters, show that even very small levels of exposure can have huge effects in offspring.[11]

A multitude of studies link not only BPA but also other chemical "outlaws"—phthalates, hexachlorocyclohexane (lindane), pentachlorophenol, DDT, atrazone, dioxins, furans, poly—chlorinated biphenyls, and some heavy metals, among others—to health threats worldwide.[12] In response to such daunting evidence, legislation has been introduced in Congress to force a federal ban on BPA.[13]

No Safety in Numbers

When it comes to BPA exposure, it's a mistake to think that the "more—is—worse—for—you" paradigm that has dominated the field of toxicology holds true—or will protect you. When chemicals that can disrupt the body's signaling systems are delivered *at the wrong time*—even in tiny amounts of parts per billion or even parts per trillion—they can have profound effects on all aspects of health. And this applies whether you're an adult, a child, or an infant.

Here's how such chemical—based "hormone havoc" can cause you to gain weight:

The endocrine system is made up of glands, hormones, and receptors that affect virtually all bodily processes: reproduction, immunity, metabolism, behavior, and organs such as the heart, ovaries, testes, and thyroid. When compounds that mimic our hormones disrupt the signals that trigger, say, estrogen metabolism and other intricate hormonal processes, then the naturally occurring timing, coordination, and delivery of hormones to cells is hijacked, amplified, or otherwise distorted.

The effects of such hormonal havoc can be far—reaching. Not only might you be prone to weight gain, but your reproduction system, brain development, behavior, temperature, and other body functions could be affected. Endocrine disruptors could injure or destroy a hormone—producing organ such as the thyroid, which regulates your "baseline" (basal) metabolic rate—making it even harder for you to lose weight and keep it off.[14]

Obesogens, Chemical Cuisine, and Your Weight

Are such concerns justified? The answer is a resounding "yes"—because BPA and its many chemical cousins (pesticides, herbicides, phthalates found in some cosmetics and soft plastic toys, etc.) can create havoc with our hormones. Theo Colburn coined the term "endocrine disruptors" (EDs)[10] to describe man—made chemicals that have the power to function as *synthetic* hormones throughout the body (see the sidebar "No Safety in Numbers") and, in turn, threaten health and affect the way fat is distributed in your body.

Have you had your endocrine disruptors today? Probably. About seven billion pounds of BPA are produced globally every year, and all of us are probably infused with it in varying amounts.[16] The body gets rid of BPA pretty quickly, so the levels detected in population studies show that we are constantly ingesting BPA.

Ongoing exposure is worrisome not only because of the many ailments linked to the ingestion of BPA and other EDs, but also because a growing number of researchers are exploring how these man−made chemicals can trigger striking increases in body fat.[10] The BPA−obesity link is considered so pervasive that biologist Bruce Blumberg of the University of California, Irvine, has coined the word "obesogens" to describe the eighty−plus identified artificial compounds that can contribute to weight gain. [17,18] (See the sidebar "Chemicals that Can Cause Obesity.")

Chemicals that Can Cause Obesity

BPA and other endocrine disruptors that mimic the hormone estrogen are of particular concern because estrogen receptors are "promiscuous"—they mate with many different estrogen−like molecules. Such "promiscuity" makes humans susceptible to a wide range of estrogen−like pollutants, including the following:

- **Estrogens** (DES, bisphenol−A, genistein)
- **Phthalates** (monobutyryl phthalate, DEHP)
- **Organochlorines** (atrazine, trans−nonachlor, oxychlordane)
- **Dioxins and polychlorinated biphenyls**
- **Organotins** (tributyltin, triphenyltin)

According to Blumberg, "It makes a lot of sense that chemicals able to reprogram metabolism and favor the development of fat cells could be important contributing factors to obesity."[19] Here's how Dr. Mehmet Oz describes obesogens and the ways in which they wreak havoc on your weight:

There's a new group of secret saboteurs in the war against weight gain. They're called obesogens, and they are all around us .... These natural and man–made chemicals work by altering the regulatory system that controls our weight—increasing the fat cells you have, decreasing the calories you burn, and even altering the way your body manages hunger .... By mimicking the actions of naturally occurring hormones in our bodies or preventing the hormones we produce from acting correctly, endocrine disruptors can:

• Encourage the body to store fat and re–program cells to become fat cells.

• Prompt the liver to become insulin resistant, which makes the pancreas pump out more insulin that turns energy into fat all over the body.

• Prevent leptin (a hormone that reduces appetite) from being released from your fat cells to tell your body you are full.

Where do you find obesogens? The short answer: everywhere. For example, high fructose corn syrup, which can be found in almost every kind of food "product," from sodas to yogurt to pretzels, is an obesogen. The ubiquitous, viscous sweet stuff makes your liver insulin–resistant and tampers with leptin to increase your hunger, setting up a vicious cycle where you crave more food that is then more easily turned into fat. The end result: your whole body pays a hefty price by developing more body fat. [20]

Whether you use the term "endocrine disruptors" or "obesogens," the outcome of consuming what we are calling "chemical cuisine" is the same: these unwelcome substances hijack your body's metabolic setpoints. In this way, the odds skyrocket that you'll accumulate body fat and become overweight.[21]

Programmed to be Fat?

The chemical cuisine/weight gain equation may seem simple: con—sume obesogens through food, beverages, or the air you breathe, and you're likely to gain weight. But the impact of these stealthy chemi—cals is even more insidious than that. Yes, evidence from many labora—tories has shown that even low doses of a variety of EDs can promote weight gain and obesity.[17] But many of these studies have been done on animals such as mice. The question of whether they can actually harm humans remained unanswered . . . until quite recently.

In 2004, T. Takeuchi and colleagues in Japan conducted one of the first studies that linked BPA to human health and weight. When the researchers compared BPA levels in normal—weight and obese women, those who were obese had significantly higher blood levels of BPA. This same study showed that women with polycystic ova—ries also had much higher blood levels of BPA than healthy control subjects.[22] More recent research has linked exposure to BPAs to both heart disease and diabetes.[23]

Such studies prompt this question: if consumption of BPA is linked to obesity and other health—robbing conditions in adults, what might happen when babies are fed canned formula containing BPA, in BPA—laden plastic bottles? How might undeveloped digestive sys—tems and fat cells respond to an onslaught of obesogens from pesticides in soy formula (used by about 20 percent of American mothers)—chemicals ranging from herbicides and fungicides to insecticides and bactericides intended for preventing, destroying, or controlling pests that could interfere with food production?[1, 24,25]

In 2005, the year after Japanese researchers found a connec—tion between blood BPA levels and obesity in adults, scientists in Spain looked closely at the impact of pesticides on children exposed as fetuses. The connection was clear: the more pesticides to which children were exposed in the womb, the greater their risk of being overweight as toddlers. Similar results surfaced in January 2008 when Belgian researchers found that the greater the exposure by pregnant mothers to PCBs (chemical endocrine disruptors known as chlo—rinated hydrocarbons, used in hundreds of products until they were banned in 1979) and DDE (the chemical byproduct of the pesticide DDT), the more obese their children were.[26]

While such findings are a cause for concern, developmental reproductive biologist and BPA expert Retha Newbold is quick to point out these studies don't necessarily prove that obesogen chemicals consumed by pregnant mothers cause obesity in their children. What we can conclude, though, is that the more a fetus is exposed to obesogens, the more *likely* it is that the baby will become an obese child. Endocrinologist Robert Lustig of UCSF posits that fetuses exposed to abundant obesogens have more fat cells, called *adipocytes*—and "the more adipocytes, the fatter you are."[26] But the destructive obesogen dynamic doesn't stop there. These fat-making factories are also believed to increase appetite and activate the brain hormones that make us feel hungry. Combine being born with a lot of fat cells and feeling hungry, and your body's been set up for overeating, gaining weight, and hanging onto it.

Quit Chemical Cuisine!

Given that BPA and other chemical compounds linked with obesity have made their way into many parts of our lives, getting them out of our diet is a daunting endeavor. Still, you can turn around a sense of defeatism by taking positive action to protect yourself. Here are some simple steps for avoiding an ongoing onslaught of these unwelcome substances.

Be Food-Wise

Go organic. Organically produced foods are made without obesogens such as antibiotics and synthetic hormones. In our book about how food resets genes for wellness or illness, we offer this advice from cookbook author Jay Weinstein: "To find out if produce without the USDA organic seal is organic . . . [check] the Product Look Up Code (PLU) on produce stickers: four digits means it's not organic; if the first number is nine, then it is organic; if the number is preceded by the number eight, it has been genetically modified."[27]

Organics: Obesogen-Free Food

During the last two decades, organic farmers Carol Ann Sayle and her husband, Larry Butler, have caught the attention of thousands of fresh–food lovers with Boggy Creek Farm in Austin, Texas, which they describe as their "USDA–certified–organic urban market farm."

Carol Ann and Larry irrigate their farm, named after a nearby creek, from a centuries–old well. Customers who visit on market days—Wednesdays and Saturdays—rhapsodize about the beau–tiful, taste–filled, chemical–free vegetables Boggy Creek pro–duces. Carol Ann, who is also an artist, views her vegetables with an aesthetic sensibility that threads its way through the placement of the crops in the fields to the arrangement of the vegetables on the market tables. Reaping the rewards of this flavor–filled canvas asks us to take the time to see and savor both the visible and invisible ingredients that go into making the produce that unequivocally nourishes body, mind, and soul.

When we recently spoke to Carol Ann, she had the following things to say about her operation. For more about Carol Ann's and Larry's innovative organic farm and day–to–day "News of the Farm," visit their website (www.boggycreekfarm.com).

In the beginning. "Because nothing with chemicals had ever been done to our farmland, it was fairly easy to get certified as an organic farm when we officially began in 1994. Back then, organic vegetables were a new idea, so we often had to explain what we *didn't* do: no chemicals or herbicides. We also talked about how we care for our soil. At the time, organic fertilizer didn't exist, so we added cow manure and used our trees to feed and nourish the soil. Even without using chemicals, our produce thrived."

Fresh is best. "Our whole premise is to eat in season because that's your best chance of getting fresh food, which is equally as important as organic in terms of flavor and quality, in that fresh, seasonal vegetables are brimming with vitamins, minerals, anti–

oxidants, phytonutrients, and so on. A fresh experience is what we're going for at Boggy Creek, so people will get as much nutrition from our food as possible."

Nourishing body, mind, soul. "I know our food is filled with vitality and the life force, because I've walked in my fields and approached my plants at night when the moon is out. During this time, I've felt the energy, the quivering of the plants; they're very alive. And it's this life–giving energy we want to eat, meaning that when the vegetable plants are in the ground, they're alive. You'll get all the life force from the vegetable if you eat it from the ground as soon as possible. After all, this is how humans ate for tens of thousands of years.

"It's beautiful to see the miracle of life happening on the farm, to see seeds germinate and then come up. It's also gratifying to feed the crop good, healthy food and soil, so that people who eat our vegetables can be well nourished. Over the years, customers have told me they have more energy when they eat our food; that it nurtures their body, brain, *and* soul."

Attitude of gratitude. "The miracle of food, the community, the nourishment, the delight . . . it's a circle and it's all connected. I thank the people who come to Boggy Creek Farm on market days. They make it possible for Larry and me to continue to do what we love."[28]

Get wild. Because of what's in its feed, *farm-raised* salmon is one of the most contaminated protein sources of polychlorinated biphenyls; indeed, farm–raised fish has up to ten times the amount of this toxic industrial pollutant as wild salmon. Another reason to "go wild": although farmed salmon has high levels of health–friendly omega–3 fatty acids, it has even higher amounts of health–harming omega–6 fatty acids.[29]

Be fresh. As often as possible, choose fresh, whole food in its natural state. While organic is optimal, fresh or frozen fruits and vegetables are preferable to produce sold in cans (see "Kick the Cans," below.

Wash well. To reduce exposure to pesticides, wash fruits and veg‐etables in organic solutions available in many supermarkets. At the least, always rinse with water.

Choose lean. Many obesogens are stored in the fat of animal foods—meat, poultry, eggs, dairy (cheese, milk, ice cream, yogurt, and so on). To reduce exposure, choose low‐fat, lean foods as often as possible. Avoid highly processed meat products, such as bologna or smoked ham, because they tend to be high in fat and chemicals.

Be butcher-friendly. Prepackaged meat in the supermarket con‐tains BPA because of its plastic packaging. Instead, opt to buy meats directly from the butchers in the meat department—and ask them to wrap your purchase in paper.

Kick the cans. Most tin cans have linings with BPA‐filled epoxy resin. Avoid canned foods and instead opt for products in glass con‐tainers. Another option: tuna in pouches that don't contain BPA.

Be natural. If organic isn't an option, seek out foods labeled "nat‐ural." While the definition of "natural" remains somewhat vague, foods labeled as such seem to be minimally processed and "less bad for you" than conventionally processed food. Here how the Food Marketing Institute (FMI) defines "natural":

> The term "natural" applies broadly to foods that are minimally processed and free of synthetic preservatives; artificial sweeteners, colors, flavors, and other artificial additives; growth hormones; antibiotics; hydrogenated oils; stabilizers; and emulsifiers. Most foods labeled natural are not subject to government controls beyond the regulations and health codes that apply to all foods. Exceptions include meat and poultry.[30]

Stay cool. Obesogens can be released when food in plastic con−
tainers is heated in a microwave oven or when hot food touches
plastic wrap. The implication is clear: don't let hot food come in con−
tact with plastic.

Be Beverage-Wise

Shun BPA-bottles. BPA has been banned from baby bottles, but
it's still present in many other plastic products, especially sports water
bottles, food packaging, and canned colas.

- Choose glass, stainless−steel, or BPA−free aluminum water con−
  tainers whenever possible.

- Warm temperatures increase the odds of BPA leaching. Don't keep
  plastic bottles in your car, where they can get quite warm.

- When plastic bottles are your only option, be "number−smart" (see
  below).

Get number-smart. BPA−free plastic wat
er bottles and baby bottles are getting easier to find all the time. To
lower the odds of getting BPA−laden bottles, select plastic numbered
1, 2, 4, 5, or 6. Plastic bottles with the number 3 or 7 on the bottom
might leach BPA.

Filter your water. Place an activated carbon filter on your water
faucet to filter out unwanted obesogen chemicals, such as atrazine
(see "Filter Faucets," below).

Be Kitchen-Wise

Avoid plastic. Besides BPA, many plastic containers contain poly−
vinylchloride (vinyl or PVC), described by researcher Paul Goettlich,
who writes about the effects of technology on our bodies, as a "health
hazard from production through disposal" and "a worst plastic for any

purpose."[31] To avoid PVC, choose glass or stainless−steel food pack−aging, cookware and utensils, and storage containers. Some possibili−ties: milk in glass bottles; glass spice and jam jars; stainless−steel mixing bowls, colanders, canteens, bottles, measuring cups, and spoons.

Filter faucets. Because pesticides seep into soil, it's possible they'll find their way to your tap water. Two culprit obesogens in tap water are atrazine (banned in Europe but abundant in the United States, it slows metabolism) and tributylin (a fungicide that stimulates fat cell production).[32] When cooking, use filtered water from the faucet.

No nonstick. In animal studies, research has shown that prenatal exposure to the chemical perfluorooctanoic acid (PFOA)—used to make Teflon pans, Gore−Tex clothing, and non−stain carpets—leads to elevated insulin levels and obesity in later life. [33] Another possible threat to your weight: PFOA affects thyroid glands, which produce weight−regulating hormones, and may be implicated in thyroid dis−ease.[23] If your Teflon pan gets scratched, toss it, because a scratch on the surface can release the chemicals inside. PFOA is also concealed in microwave popcorn bags and pizza boxes. As much as possible, avoid food and household products that might contain PFOA.

Be Home-Wise

Reject vinyl. Phthalates found in vinyl flooring, plastic shower cur−tains, and industrial−grade plastic wrap could lower testosterone and metabolism levels, causing you to gain weight and lose muscle mass. Choose non−vinyl flooring such as ceramic tile or wood, hang nylon or cotton shower curtains, and have your meat wrapped in brown paper at the grocery store.

Breathe real air. Phthalates are also found in air fresheners. Choose natural oils to scent your home, or simply open your windows or doors every day to air out your home.

Take Control

Ultimately, the message in our "quit chemical cuisine" guidelines is simple: you can help make weight loss last by making conscious anti−obesogen choices about food and beverages. Every time you shop for, prepare, and eat food, you are empowered to reduce your exposure to obesogens and live a weight−smart life.

Regardless of your age—five months, five years, fifty, or older—the invisible and unwelcome "nutrients" known as obesogens can invade your body and make you more apt to overeat and gain weight. But putting on extra pounds doesn't have to be your fate if you take action now.

Chapter 10

Sleep More, Weigh Less

Plenty of weight–loss products promise miracles. We recall one in particular that promised a magic pill to let you lose weight while you sleep. But what if you don't need a mystical (and questionable) potion to lose weight while sleeping? What if all you need to increase the chances of losing weight—and making weight loss last—is sleep itself? Can you think of an easier way to lose weight?

There are two caveats. First, you need to sleep enough hours to reap the benefits. If you skimp on sleep, the converse occurs: you're more likely to put on pounds. Second, our message throughout this book still holds: it's a combined effort. Losing weight and keeping it off means making lasting lifestyle changes that include the solutions we've discussed so far along with sleeping soundly more often than not.

Counting Zzzs

Are you really more prone to put on pounds when you don't get enough sleep? Absolutely, says Sanjay Patel, lead investigator of a study that added the issue of inadequate sleep to the obesity landscape in 2006. To come to this unexpected conclusion, Dr. Sanjay R. Patel, Division of Pulmonary and Critical Care Medicine, Case Western Reserve University, and his team conducted the largest–ever sleep study of its kind. Starting in 1986, they undertook a sixteen–year study that would track the sleep habits of almost 70,000 middle–aged women nurses. But they did more than merely observe sleep routines:

the researchers linked the number of hours each woman slept each night to her weight over time.

What Patel found was remarkable: about 33 percent of the women who slept five hours or less per night each gained thirty−three pounds or more over the course of the study, while an additional 15 percent gained even more and became obese. In comparison, 12 percent of the women who slept one hour longer each night—an average of six hours—were also likely to gain weight, but less so: only 6 percent become obese. And then the good news emerged: those who typi−cally managed seven hours or more nightly gained the least weight.

Patel's study yielded three especially intriguing insights. The first is that the sleep less/weigh more link was there when the study started: women who slept five hours or less nightly already averaged about 5.4 pounds more in weight than those who managed at least seven hours each night. The second finding further verified the con−nection, in that over a ten−year time span, the more sleep−deprived women gained an average of 1.6 pounds each year. While this may not seem like much, over a period of ten years it could mean sixteen added pounds—or, if the trend held, a gain of thirty−two pounds over twenty years. The third insight is the bottom line of Patel's study: women who sleep five hours or less each night are 32 percent more likely to put on weight than those who sleep seven hours or more.[1]

Were Patel's findings a fluke? Or did his sixteen−year study uncover a new clue about why so many of us find it difficult to lose weight and, if we do, to keep it off? Over the next few years, several good studies on the sleep−weight connection, conducted with all age groups in several countries, confirmed Patel's findings: there *is* a cor−relation between how much you sleep and how much you weigh. But the lesson of the sleep−weight link suggests even more: the mind−body is exquisitely sensitive to the *quality* of sleep. Sleeping too little, too much, or just enough may create chemical changes throughout your mind−body that tip the weight scale up . . . or down.[2-4]

The Sleep Less Life

If you find it difficult to get to sleep or to stay asleep, you have a lot of company: about seventy million Americans are affected by chronic sleep loss.[5] In fact, insufficient sleep is a growing problem in modern society. Over the past fifty years, the average number of hours we sleep each night has decreased by two hours; and from 1998 to 2005, the percentage of those getting eight hours of sleep dropped from 36 percent to 25 percent.[6]

There are lots of reasons for not getting enough sleep. When you go to bed, do you worry about work, say, or money? Or do you watch TV or surf the Web well into the wee hours? Not only may such behaviors make you anxious or depressed, but light from TV and computer monitors that stimulates the brain can also wreak havoc with your natural sleep cycle. Or perhaps you've developed a full-blown sleeping disorder (see the sidebar "Sleep Problems that Can Cause Weight Gain").

Sleep Problems that Can Cause Weight Gain

Most of us have had trouble falling asleep at some time, then feeling sleepy the next day. But if tossing and turning becomes a common occurrence, you may be suffering from a sleep disorder. This matters a lot, because ongoing poor-quality sleep causes more than just fatigue, irritability, and a sense of sleepiness and low energy; it can affect both your physical health (weight gain, diabetes, high blood pressure) and your emotional well-being (depression, anxiety). Here are some common sleep problems.

Insomnia occurs when you find it hard to fall or stay asleep throughout the night. If this happens only occasionally, you may have acute (also called *transient*) insomnia; if it happens a lot, you could have chronic insomnia.

Sleep apnea is a condition wherein you actually stop breathing while asleep. It occurs when soft tissues in the back of the throat and neck relax so much that the airway narrows or even gets blocked completely, preventing air from getting through. Struggling to breath, the body briefly wakes up—even if the person doesn't realize it.[7,8] If someone is overweight, especially in the neck area, sleep apnea is more likely to be serious. Of special concern is the fact that most of the twenty–two million Americans who have this debilitating condition don't know it.[9]

Narcolepsy is characterized by excessive daytime sleepiness, sudden attacks of muscular weakness (cataplexy), and a strong need to sleep. About 50 percent of adults with this disorder report symptoms starting in the teen years.[10]

Circadian rhythm sleep disorders are linked with the body's biological "clock" (circadian rhythms). Sleep affects circadian rhythms, which in turn affect your body temperature, alertness, appetite, hormone secretion, and sleep timing. Your body's natu–rally occurring rhythm can be influenced in a number of ways. A sampling:

• *Jet lag* strikes when the body's circadian rhythms are altered due to travelling across several time zones.

• *Shift work sleep disorder* affects people who work nights or rotating shifts.

• *Delayed sleep phase disorder* (DSPD) manifests itself with peak alertness in the middle of the night.

• *Advanced sleep phase syndrome* (ASPS) is characterized by dif–ficulty staying awake in the evening and difficulty staying asleep in the morning.

• *Non-24*, or non–24–hour sleep–wake syndrome, describes a sleep pattern that occurs later and later each day.

• *Irregular sleep-wake rhythm* refers to sleeping at irregular times, such as taking many naps during the day.

In the "Sleep More, Weigh Less" section of this chapter, we suggest strategies for lowering the likelihood of having a sleep disorder, and we offer guidelines for sleeping well so that you can make weight loss last—even while asleep.

Full−blown sleeping disorders and unhealthy sleep−related behaviors may not be the only reason for sleeplessness. For the 67 percent of women who experience some kind of sleep problem, there may be other causes. One culprit seems to be the hormonal mix that occurs after first pregnancy through menopause (that is, between twenty−something and fifty−something). During this time, hormone shifts can lead to mood switches from calmness to high−pitched anxiety. The hormone link? Naturally occurring low levels of progesterone especially can lead to a sense of "being on edge."

Especially with first−borns, but with infants and small children in general, sleep deprivation is a sometimes−overwhelming fact of parenting life. A colicky infant can mean that you never get more than a snatched nap for weeks on end. Even when children are older, sleep interruptions are an ordinary part of child−rearing. These patterns can go on long enough to disrupt "normal" sleep for years. Add the "you−can−have−it−all" sensibility that permeates our culture, and women especially have a recipe for sleeplessness . . . and weight gain.

Sleep Studies and Your Weight

The sleep more/weigh less formula may seem simple, but a closer look reveals the picture isn't quite so black and white. Population−based sleep studies such as Sanjay Patel's 16−year project don't establish definitively that lack of sleep causes obesity. Such studies strongly suggest there may be something to the formula, but an apparent link (called a "correlation" in science) doesn't necessarily mean that lack of sleep actually *causes* weight gain.

But there does seem to be some kind of connection, and that leads to this question: is poor sleep an actual contributor to today's obesity epidemic? To find out, researchers have looked closely at mechanisms by which sleep loss may lead to obesity. Here are some of their theories:

Less exercise. When you don't sleep well, energy levels ebb and you feel fatigue.[11] In turn, when you're tired, you're less likely to exercise. Even if you're not an exerciser, fatigue may mean you don't move around as much as when you've sleep well. Any kind of move—ment—from fidgeting to a full—blown workout—burns calories, while moving less conserves energy, so the less—exercise theory states that sleepiness may lead to more stored fat and obesity. Still, when researchers adjusted for exercise in the lack—of—sleep and obesity equation, whether a person exercised or not didn't play a part.[1,2]

More snacking. Do shift work, late—night TV or internet surfing, and access to stores 24/7 give us more chances to snack and thus increase caloric intake?[12] The answer is yes. When you're sleep deprived, you're more likely to reach for the carrot cake instead of the carrot, to want high—calorie carbohydrates (such as cake and ice cream) and high—fat foods (such as fried chicken and burgers).[13] Why is that? When researchers showed images of food to people who were well rested versus sleep deprived, the area of the brain that controls appetite (the anterior cingulated cortex) lit up in the sleep—deprived individuals, not so for their well—rested counterparts. In other words, when sleep—deprived individuals see high—calorie foods, a part of their brain becomes excited.[14] In this way, sleepiness may lead to overeating and, in turn, to weight gain.

Brain-hormone link. It's not just the sleep—deprived *brain* that gets turned on at the sight of high—calorie food (see "More snacking," above). Sleep loss may also activate *hormones* that can amp up the urge to eat. It works like this: inadequate sleep decreases leptin, the hormone that turns *off* your appetite; at the same time, sleep loss increases the appetite—*stimulating* hormone ghrelin.[13] This one—two hormone punch leads to more food consumption, especially when too little sleep launches the brain—activated preference for high—fat, high—carbohydrate food.

And there's a "knockout" to the one—two hormone punch: when you're sleep deprived, even if hormones don't lead to overeating, your mood may take you there. Not getting enough sleep is associated with unpleasant feelings—from irritability and impatience to pessimism, fatigue, and stress[15]—that are likely to turn your attention to "comfort foods" and "feel good" treats such as chocolate as a way to feel better.[16] Add these unpleasant moods to a reduced resolve to exercise and a craving for high−fat food, and you have yet another formula for overeating and weight gain.

Slower metabolism. Metabolism is the naturally occurring bio−chemical activity by which food is converted into energy to main−tain the body. Some studies have shown that when you don't get enough sleep, your metabolism slows down and your core tempera−ture drops.[17] When this happens, the speed at which you burn calories is impaired; therefore, it's easier to put on pounds. What's especially telling about these findings is this: *even if you cut calories and exercise, if your metabolism slows because you're sleep deprived, you're still likely to gain weight.*[18, 19] In other words, to lose weight when you're sleep deprived, you need to increase your metabolism by exercising *more*. Sleep well and you'll need less exercise.

Daylight saving time savvy. The simple ritual of resetting clocks one hour forward or back takes on new meaning with a study that showed how daylight saving time—a seemingly small change—affects sleep performance in teens. When researchers at Rensselaer Polytechnic Institute in Troy, New York, looked at the impact increased natural light exposure in spring has on eighth graders, they found that more evening daylight repressed the buildup of the natu−rally occurring hormone melatonin. As recorded in sleep logs kept by the students, they were falling asleep an average of sixteen minutes later than usual and sleeping about fifteen minutes less than during the winter.

Even sixteen minutes less sleep can make a big difference in well−being, because when it gets dark outside, melatonin sends signals throughout the body telling you it's time to get ready for sleep. The gradual buildup of melatonin usually precedes falling asleep by several hours. But with the *sudden* extra hour of daylight (meaning that the internal clock hasn't had time to adjust to the change), teens stayed up later and got less sleep—so much so that they experienced mood changes and poor academic performance, and likely risked increased weight gain as well.[20] (For more about melatonin, light levels, and sleep, see "Discover the light side of dark" section.)

Sleep More, Weigh Less

The dozens of sleep–weight studies that have been done with different populations in many countries tell us that the link between lost sleep and obesity isn't likely to be just a coincidence. These studies suggest that sleeping well is a necessity if you want to lose weight and keep it off.

From late–night Web surfing and TV watching to work worries and full–blown sleep disorders, though, there are many reasons for poor sleep habits. Luckily, there are ways to work on the problem of too little sleep. If you're a tosser and turner and want to maintain a stable and healthy body weight—to feel better and be healthier—here are some minor modifications you can make to bring major benefits.

Know your "sleep number." It's official: you can fight fat with sleep. But how much sleep does it take? Five hours? Six? Seven or more? Sleep scientists have long sought to pinpoint the optimal sleep time for healthy adults. Now researchers at West Virginia University believe they've found the "magic number": after studying 30,000 adults, they determined that seven hours is needed to avoid heart disease, heart attack, or stroke. Sleep more or fewer than seven hours, and your risk for cardiovascular disease increases.[21]

How might this translate into a general guideline for us? The American Academy of Sleep Medicine recommends that most adults get between seven and eight hours of sleep each night.[22] This range also fits into Sanjay Patel's study, which showed that women who sleep seven hours or more are less likely to be overweight.[1]

To increase your chances of getting seven and a half hours of sleep nightly, write down the time you typically wake up in the morning. Then count backward seven and a half hours. For instance, if you usually wake at 7 AM, seven and a half hours earlier would be 11:30

PM. This is the best time for you to go to sleep to ensure yourself of seven and a half hours of sleep each night.[23]

Be caffeine-free after lunch. Caffeine from soft drinks, coffee, tea, chocolate, or other beverages and foods can stay in your system hours after you've consumed it. To "de-stimulate" well in advance of your sleeping time, avoid consuming caffeine-containing products after lunch.

Avoid alcohol within six hours of bedtime. Most of us think of alcoholic beverages (wine, beer, vodka, and so on) as relaxing, so it may be a surprise to discover that imbibing too close to sleep time can actually keep you awake.

Create a Relaxing Bedtime Routine

Establishing a regular routine, perhaps an hour or so before bed-time, is a great aid in getting a good night's sleep. Choose strate-gies you know will work well for you. Here are a few possibilities.

- Take a warm bath.
- Listen to calming music.
- Put soothing, scented oil (such as lavender) on sore muscles and gently massage the area for a few minutes.

Practice any other relaxation techniques in this section that reso-nate with you.

Sip something soothing. Try naturally relaxing herbal teas to enhance sleep. Some have a calming effect on the nervous system: lemon balm, lavender, linden, chamomile, valerian, and passion flower.

Pause worry-filled thoughts. Is this scenario familiar to you? Feeling sleepy, you go to bed at 11 PM. But the moment you switch off the light and your head hits the pillow, stress-filled thoughts start. Is my job secure? What can I do about my credit-card debt? What if I mess up tomorrow's presentation? Instead of ruminating over such "what ifs," keep a notepad on your nightstand and write down your worries before turning off the light. Just list them. Then decide on a specific time the next day to think about your list. Schedule fifteen to thirty minutes for your worry session.

Turn off the TV and computer monitor. Watching TV before going to sleep can slow down getting to sleep in these two ways: (1) the light from the screen can diminish production of sleep−inducing melatonin, the hormone your body produces when it gets dark; and (2) your brain is stimulated by TV stories, dialogue, and often−loud music (especially during commercials). The double−whammy of light and brain stimulation can curtail sleep. To sleep well, turn off your TV and your computer about an hour before it's time to sleep.

Avoid exercising close to bedtime. Regular exercise in the morning or early afternoon is preferable to exercise close to sleep time, because exercising energizes your body.

Reset your body's biological clock. One of the most useful steps you can take to ensure a good night's sleep, *each night*, is to maintain a regular bedtime and waking time—weekends included.

Be sleepy. The idea of being sure you're sleepy before going to bed may seem obvious. We're bringing it up because if you go to bed because you "should" rather than because your mind−body is ready for a good night's sleep, you're likely to toss and turn. Not feeing sleepy may be a particular problem during daylight saving time. The solution: go to bed earlier when the clock "springs forward" in spring, later when time "falls backward" in autumn.

Enhance your bedroom atmosphere. There's a lot you can do to create an environment that encourages sleep. For example:

• Be sure your mattress is comfortable.

• Use your bedroom solely for sleep (or sex).

• Choose sheets and blankets that "welcome" you with colors and texture you like.

Sleep cool. Staying cool throughout the night enhances sleep. Some cool strategies:

• Keep the bedroom temperature slightly cool.

• Select a mattress pad made of natural fabric, such as cotton, so that it "breathes." Mattress pads, sheets, pillow cases, or blankets made of synthetic fabrics (such as polyester) can lock in moisture and make you so warm that you wake up.

• For a sleep–enhancing treat that keeps your body temperature stable while you sleep, consider a Feel Cooler cooling mattress pad. It's so effective, it's used by astronauts.

Discover the light side of dark. Exposure to light while sleeping can cause levels of the sleep–friendly hormone melatonin to decline quickly. This can interrupt the sleep cycle, even if you don't awake fully. Make your bedroom as free of light as possible with dense cur–tains and alarm clocks that don't directly "glare" at you. Consider wearing an eye mask that blocks out light.

Get quiet. Unwelcome sounds or full–blown noise can keep you awake. To achieve quiet and sleep more soundly, use earplugs—or try a sound machine that creates "white noise" to block out other noise.

Make Up for Lost Sleep?

Is it really possible to make up for lost sleep? Sort of. After lead researcher David Dinges of the University of Pennsylvania School of Medicine severely restricted the sleep of 142 adults for five days, allowing only four hours of sleep nightly, study participants recovered to various degrees. How they felt depended on the number of hours of "recovery sleep" they got—how long they spent sleeping after being deprived of sleep. Those who slept about ten hours recovered best; those with the fewest hours of sleep experienced less recovery.

So, can you really make up for lost sleep? You may feel somewhat better after "sleeping in," but according to Dinges, sleep debt remained even after a night of extended sleep.[24]

Feed your brain. It's possible that if you're not sleeping well, the food you are eating—or not eating—may be playing a part. Sleeping through the night depends on providing the brain with adequate amounts of fuel energy in the form of glucose. Undereat, and your brain may not get enough glucose to help you sleep through the night. In response, your body produces the fight–or–flight hormone cortisol, which can keep you awake.

To keep glucose levels stable—both during the day and at night—eat breakfast soon after getting up, have lunch about four hours afterward, then eat a light dinner between 6 and 7 PM. If you haven't eaten a snack or dinner three to four hours before going to bed, try calming carbohydrates and health–filled fat, such as an apple with a teaspoon or so of nut butter (peanut, sesame/tahini, almond, or cashew, for example) to encourage sleep.

Breath deeply. Here's a quick and easy three–step strategy than can lead to restful sleep. Do these steps slowly, three to five times.

1. Inhale deeply to the count of 5.
2. Hold your breath to the count of 2.
3. Exhale to the count of 7.

See a sleep specialist. For many, changing their nighttime habits and practicing good sleep hygiene gives them the rest–filled sleep they want. For others, such strategies may not be enough. You don't have to continue suffering if sleep problems persist. Instead, see a sleep doctor. These specialists are trained to pinpoint the cause of your sleeplessness and will work with you to find the remedy. They can help you with a weight–loss plan as well, if needed, because obesity is often linked with sleep issues.

Sleep: A Necessity, Not a Luxury

On the surface, it seems so simple: get a good night's sleep and you're more likely to make weight loss last. Of course, a good night's sleep isn't always so simple to implement. The demands of home, family, and career—and the lure of technology—make it challenging to carve out quality sleep time. Once you learn the healing possibilities of sleep, though, health problems—from gaining weight, blood pressure, and mood, to diabetes, and more—may be prevented or at the least, better managed.[25] Given such benefits, sleep is a necessity, not a luxury.

Chapter 11

Get Moving

In the first chapter of this book, we described the solutions in *Make Weight Loss Last* as a way of life, a "whole person" approach to nutrition and eating that nourishes your biological, psychological, spiritual, and social well–being. If your intention is to lose weight and you stay with it, we wrote, you'll accomplish that, and much more: you'll enjoy more balanced emotions, spiritual well–being, and social connection.

So, too, with motion. Look up the word "motion," and you'll find it described as "movement," "action," and "activity." Or "exer–cise," "training," and "workout." Whichever way you turn the kinetic kaleidoscope, exercise heals you physically, emotionally, spiritually, and socially. And by burning calories and speeding up your metabo–lism, it helps you stay slim.

Because motion has this power to heal multidimensionally, *and* to make weight loss last, we are including this chapter about ways to "get moving." How do our guidelines differ from more traditional exer–cise? As with the solutions to the seven overeating styles, the answer is both simple and profound: through an understanding and apprecia–tion of how movement impacts your *entire being*.

Four-Facet Exercise for the Whole Person
Not long ago a friend named Bruce Heller told us how his passion for movement began. "It became part of my life when I began to ride my bike to elementary school. By biking to school, to after–school activities, and to friends' homes, or to just hang out, I wasn't

dependent on my parents to drive me places, so over time, riding my bike came to symbolize a sense of freedom and independence. When I was a teenager, I started to ride my bicycle with other kids in the neighborhood. Now, as an adult, I ride my mountain bike as a stress—relieving activity; I do it for hours as a way to relax and stay in shape."

Heller is a family physician who is passionate about food and nutrition, exercise, and health. A specialist in integrative medicine who uses both Western and Eastern healing practices to prevent and treat obesity and related ailments, from heart disease and high blood pressure to diabetes, Heller first looks at lifestyle interven—tions to help his patients. Exercise plays a central role because not only does it influence his patients' physiology, helping to prevent and reverse health conditions, but it also influences mood, well—being, and overall vitality. "We were made to move," says Heller. "Human beings evolved as moving animals."

Realizing that exercise holds the power to heal in every way, Heller integrates it into his holistic healing recommendations to patients; it's also an integral part of his own life, a way to balance the demands of a busy practice. During a recent conversation, Heller shared a particu—larly memorable "whole person" exercise experience from his days as a medical resident, when he often worked 100—hour weeks:

I used to call Annadel State Park in Santa Rosa, California, my church. During residency when I was busy and sleep deprived, often the only time I would have for a major workout was Sunday mornings at Annadel. I would wake up anticipating my mountain bike ride. Because my life was so busy and I had so little time, taking off on my bike brought back the sense of freedom and independence I had experienced as a youth on my bicycle. But now bike rides were even more meaningful because they were augmented by my appreciation of the beauty of nature, which has always been where I go to recharge. I look forward not only to moving my body, but also to being outside in a beautiful place surrounded by nature. For me, pine trees represent cathedral spires, and there is a contemplative quality to a redwood forest—quite a contrast to the hours I spent indoors as a resident, working long, late hours in a busy hospital, caring for sick people, often sur—rounded by life—or—death situations.

To balance this, I would start Sunday mornings with a cup of tea and gentle yoga, stretching and focusing on each position (asana) consciously and mindfully. Interestingly, even when you just anticipate exercise, your body prepares you for the activity you're about to engage in; your physiology changes in antici—pation. Even before you start running or biking or doing the activity, blood vessels dilate to bring more blood to the muscles; your heart rate speeds up to increase cardiac output; and breathing rate increases. It's almost as if you're warming up without actually warming up. Most people think exercise is purely physical, but there's also a mind—body connection. Your body knows it's going to need more blood and oxygen to power the muscles you'll be using when you move, so it starts helping you out even before you actually begin.

Annadel is a 5,200—acre park, filled with creeks, redwood groves, and meadows, and has about forty miles of trails. Entering the park on a fire road, I would ride past children and their fami—lies who were picnicking and feeding ducks, while others would be fishing in a stock pond. The higher up in elevation I would go on my mountain bike, the narrower the dirt trails would become. I especially enjoyed this because these are the most technically challenging trails: you have to be careful to avoid rocks, ruts, and roots. When I ride up and down steep inclines and declines, it gives me a strong sense of well—being and accomplishment. With a sigh of relief, I appreciate that I've made it to the top. My body feels good. When I'm riding my bike, focused and concentrating on the terrain in front of me, I'm not always able to appreciate nature. But at the top of the ridge, it's all around me. I can see it all at my leisure; I'm on top of the world.

But there's more. After riding through the pine forest in the park, and then up and down two steep peaks, Heller would often reward himself toward the end of the ride with a swim in the park's lake. The total time for his exercise experience was two hours, sometimes three.

Physical Feats

When Heller started his ride, at the outset he could sense which muscles were sore, and feel any stiffness in his legs or neck. But after twenty minutes on his bike, with his blood flowing and his muscles warming, he hit his natural pace. At this stage of his ride, the terrain was still pretty mellow, with gently rolling hills. After about twenty-five minutes, he would get to his first steep incline, which meant about a mile and a half of uphill riding. To ease resistance, he would click into a lower gear, stand up on the pedals, and start working a lot harder to stay at the same speed or cadence (how fast you're spinning the pedals). His breathing would quicken, his heart would beat faster, and he would break a sweat. After about twenty minutes, he would get to the top of the hill.

Throughout the ride, Heller's body would automatically do what was necessary to give him energy for the activity: his blood vessels would dilate to bring more blood, a carrier of oxygen, to power his cells and energize his muscles. "The metabolism of your cells is like an engine," he explains. "You can be more efficient or less efficient at burning energy. If you don't exercise and you're a couch potato, your body isn't doing what it is meant to do: move. Breathing and digesting food still take energy, but your engine is running idly and inefficiently."

In contrast, every time you exercise, you have a whole body experience for your cardiovascular, musculoskeletal, respiratory, endocrine, hematologic, neurologic, and psychologic systems. You burn calories (energy) and your metabolism speeds up, you stay limber and flexible, and you build your bone density. "You burn sugar (glucose), the fuel your body uses, just the way an engine uses gasoline," says Heller. "This is especially important for diabetics, because when they exercise, their muscles use up glucose so it no longer stays in their bloodstream."

Move and be in motion five times a week for at least thirty minutes and you'll realize health benefits, including weight loss. And the benefits are ongoing: even while you're watching TV, aerobic training speeds up metabolism and burns calories. "It will make your metabolic engine run more efficiently, and burn more oxygen, which ultimately burns more glucose and allows you to lose weight," adds Heller.[1]

The Heart of Motion

Although many of us think of integrative medicine as the first whole person approach to health and healing in Western medicine, naturo—pathic medicine (sometimes called "naturopathy") has offered a com—prehensive approach to health and healing since it evolved thousands of years ago as an effective way to treat diseases. With his teaching that "nature is healer of all diseases," the Greek physician Hippocrates (c. 460 BCE–c. 370 BCE), often referred to as "the father of medicine," is thought to be the earliest naturopathic physician.

Today, modern naturopathic physicians (NDs) offer a compre—hensive system of health care based on the principle that the body tends toward health if you live according to the basic principles that govern human life—one of which is keeping the body in motion. "Every molecule, cell, tissue, and organ has a purpose," naturopathic physician Bruce Milliman told us. "All systems are geared to be engaged according to nature's design. For the natural forces of health and healing to be optimized—in muscles or joints or the brain or nervous system or blood and lymph systems or in bone and cartilage or any organ system—you have to use it or lose it."[2]

The five natural elements of Milliman's "hierarchy of necessities to live" include air, water, sleep, food, and physical activity. During the conversation with Milliman, it was the element of physical activity that particularly caught our attention, because of the unique perspec—tive he brings to it. "We have two circulatory systems," he explained. The first and primary one, the *circulatory* system—the one with which most of us are familiar—includes the heart, veins, arteries, and blood vessels. The *lymphatic* system parallels the circulatory system, but unlike the circulatory system, it doesn't have a heart. Instead, said Milliman, the heart of this second circulatory system is *physical activity, motion,* and *movement.* And it functions almost exclusively by the moving of your limbs—your arms and legs.

Consider walking. When you walk, the motion of going up and down causes the lymphatic fluids in your body to move up and down within the lymphatic system; this helps your muscles contract each time you move your limbs. All this is happening in unison with your breathing, as your diaphragm moves up and down—and as it moves, it compresses the lymphatic system, which has little valves that allow the lymph fluid to flow.

Which brings us to Milliman's second main concept ("use it or lose it" was the first)—what he calls the Black Box Theory: stuff in = stuff out + stuff stored. It's all about input and output. "Physical activity is an output," he clarified. It also integrates and balances the forces of the "use it or lose it" principle.

Put another way, because physical activity is an expression of how fit you are, it determines the degree of freedom you have in your life to be healthy and to function autonomously. When you're not fit, and if you're taking in more energy than you put out, it's likely to take different forms—such as accumulated fat, or arthritis, or swelling (edema). The concept is simple: if you don't do what you need to do (meaning, you don't do some form of motion and movement on a regular basis), your circulatory (blood) and lymphatic (lymph) systems won't function optimally. This, in turn, increases the likelihood that you'll gain weight or develop some other ailment. Motion and your physical well-being: it's all interconnected, as are exercise and your emotional well-being.[2]

Movement, Moods, and Weight

When bicyclist and physician Bruce Heller is in good shape, he welcomes the challenge of riding up steep inclines. In Annadel State Park, the trails range from gently rolling to shorter, rocky sections with steep ascents and descents. "I loved the challenge of steep and rutted trails, and trying to stay upright while going up a steep incline," he told us.

> Not only is it a great cardiovascular challenge, but it's also a technical challenge, because I have to choose a line (a term used by skiers to describe planning a path to follow) and keep my balance. Then I would feel exhilarated going downhill fast, quite a contrast to cruising through the flat redwood groves at the bottom, where it is super quiet because the abundant redwood duff on the forest floor absorbs sounds.

During the challenge of riding up and down the first steep hill, I'm concentrating on what I'm doing, and I'm completely focused on the task at hand. During this time, I'm filled with a sense of well–being, a strong feeling of accomplishment. The second major ascent and descent in the park is even steeper. As I get closer and closer to the top, I'm feeling more like I'm in the wilderness. There is no noise from cars, and I'm feeling like I've really gotten away from it all. When I get to the top, I may pause for some water or a snack. At the same time, I'm appreciating my surroundings, along with the coyotes, deer, and hawks that are often a part of it all.[3]

Exhilaration, well–being, accomplishment, appreciation: these aren't words we always associate with exercise. But if you exercise regularly, as Heller does, and you take the time to tune in to your emotions while you're in motion and when you stop, it's likely you'll be feeling pretty good. Ongoing exercise (thirty minutes or more) causes hormones (those naturally occurring chemical messengers in your body) to kick in. One of these is *endorphins*. Produced in the pituitary gland, endorphins not only *decrease your appetite*, but they also reduce tension and anxiety. Make exercise a regular part of your life, and after several months you'll experience a super high from endorphins. And they'll continue to circulate in your blood for quite a while after you've exercised.

Other hormones related to weight loss are also produced when you exercise regularly. These include *17 beta-estradiol*, the most bio–logically active estrogen, which helps break down stores of body fat so it can be used for fuel; *testosterone*, which increases your metabolism and decreases body fat; *growth hormone*, which increases the use of fat when you exercise; *thyroxine (T4)*, a hormone made by the thyroid gland that increases your metabolic rate; and *epinephrine*, a hormone produced mostly in the adrenal medulla, which stimulates stored fat to break down.

Besides the runner's high that endorphins create and the fat–burning that other hormones produce, you stand to gain even more benefits from exercise. In Chapter 4, "Access Your Appetite," we talked about emotional eating—turning to food to manage unpleasant feelings such as depression, anxiety, or anger. If you're a regular exerciser, the endorphins and other hormones you produce can replace food as your best friend when you're feeling blue. Endorphins don't just decrease your appetite: they can also reduce tension and anxiety and replace unwelcome feelings with a mild state of euphoria. Be in motion on a regular basis, and you'll be less likely to be an emotional eater.

In the Zone

"Being 'in the zone' is an indescribable experience," Heller told us. "When playing Ultimate Frisbee, I used to describe my state of mind as 'relaxed attention.' My body would be doing exactly what I wanted it to do—without my being especially attentive or focusing on it. When this happens, I have a sense of being one with the motion and my surroundings—for instance, with the bike and the trail on which I'm riding. During these times, my body knows what to do. I'm not intentionally exercising; all movement is flowing effortlessly."[4]

Many athletes describe Heller's experience of being "in the zone" in a similar way. Without conscious intention—or attention—their mind–body becomes one with the activity and environment. Somehow they're not quite in their body anymore; there's a sense that they're one with their body and the environment—and even though they may be putting out a fair amount of energy, they have a sense of effortlessness. Could it be the endorphins that have kicked in, or the alpha brain waves that combat depression and put you in a state of relaxation? Or is it a mystery, the same life force that enhances digestion and somehow stabilizes your weight when you eat with sensory regard (see Chapter 8, "Feed the Senses") and in serene surroundings (see Chapter 7, "Dine by Design")? "This spiritual connection—going in or out of the zone—can happen anytime," said Heller. "There's no way to anticipate when this is going to happen."[5]

After his bike ride in Annadel State Park, while he was feeling gratified by a challenging workout, emotionally high from the endorphins, and in the zone, Heller would often jump into the park's lake, which is in a bowl–like valley surrounded by trees. He'd end his ride by taking a quick dip to cool off. Swimming, looking at the blue sky, he'd hang out for perhaps twenty or thirty minutes, savoring the last phase of his biking adventure, the end of the ride . . . for now.

Social Fitness

When co–author Deborah first moved to San Francisco, the bus she took to her job in the financial district would pass through the city's large Chinatown district. As the bus descended the narrow, hilly, and shaded part of Sacramento Street, she would watch, transfixed, as a large group of people silently practiced *tai chi* (an ancient Chinese discipline that involves the mind, breath, and movement to create a calm, natural balance of energy) in a park in the cool morning fog. In unison and in super–slow motion, each person in the group would move through the ancient and exact movements of his or her tai chi practice. The image seemed like an oasis, something not quite real appearing suddenly and unexpectedly in the center of a major city.

Whether the activity is soccer, dance, hiking, football, bowling, or ancient Asian movements, for thousands of years people have exercised with others. As with social nutrition—dining with others instead of solo—physical activity has typically been practiced as a team activity. "I was part of the Ultimate Frisbee Team in college," Bruce Heller told us, "a group sport that's played on most college campuses. Club teams play in almost all major cities throughout the world: Europe, Africa, Asia. A lot of friends that I made twenty or more years ago when I played competitive Frisbee are still some of my best friends now. After tournaments, we would always eat out and share memories of the day. Now, as then, it's one of the most enjoyable ways to con–nect with others."[6]

Motion Possibilities

Much of *Make Weight Loss Last* focuses on eating strategies for losing weight and keeping it off. Yet the power of and exercise and optimal eating *done in unison* has been proven over and over again. One intriguing study was conducted by researchers in the Department of Kinesiology at George Washington University Medical Center in Washington, DC. To find out whether diet, aerobic exercise, or diet plus exercise brought the most weight loss, they looked at all relevant studies reported in English in peer—reviewed medical journals during the past twenty—five years. Not surprisingly, diet plus exercise tended to be the superior program for obese adults to lose weight and keep it off.[7] This tells us that physical activity is a key team member for making weight loss last.

As with the other elements we've been discussing throughout this book, integrating movement and motion into our everyday lives is yet another "way of being" from which we've veered during the last few decades. Our society has become sedentary. Television, com—puters, and video games contribute to children's inactive lifestyles; 43 percent of adolescents watch more than two hours of television each day. Children, especially girls, become less active as they progress through adolescence. The antidote? Look over the menu of move—ment options we've created for you, then follow your personal incli—nations and lifestyle needs for getting into motion.

Before you begin, we suggest that you reread the "Stages of Change" section in Chapter 2, "Jettison Judgment." This will give you insights into how to change successfully—for instance, from being a nonexer—ciser to making movement a part of your everyday life—and specific strategies for becoming a "successful loser." The mistake many of us make when we think of modifying meals and exercise is not under—standing just where we are in the Stages of Change cycle, which can tell us whether we are ready to change—really, really ready—or whether we'd benefit by first contemplating our plan. By not jumping ahead to a stage for which you may not be ready, you increase your chances of success in making exercise an integral aspect of your everyday life.

To get started, consider some of the options below. Identify the activities you resonate with the most. Think about how you can fit them into your life. Be realistic and compassionate with yourself. If you can fit in five or ten minutes, perhaps three times a day, to do something you enjoy, that's an accomplishment. "Extremercise," for hours at a time, isn't for everyone.

Follow Your "Fitness Instinct"

Medical anthropologist and fitness expert Peg Jordan has created a unique personalized approach to working out. Her philosophy: make it something you love to do, and you're more likely to succeed. To help you figure this out, Jordan has developed workout options based on what she calls your "fitness instinct," that is, ways to move based on your personal, inborn preferences and personality.

For instance, if you're a highly competitive businessperson, a stay−at−home, staid piece of equipment such as a treadmill is just going to gather dust. You're more likely to thrive playing raquetball three times a week with someone you can compete with aggressively. In contrast, Jordan offers the example of "a soccer mom who is other−directed, taking care of everybody." This person "needs to be on the buddy system for exercise," suggests Jordan, whose fitness philosophy is based on a research study. "Her best friend and she should walk together, or she should have a buddy to do swing dancing with. Exercise for this type should be social."

"Get-Going" Suggestions

Here are some of fitness expert Peg Jordan's ideas for activities to match four different "mindsets."

When you're tired...
Play with a hoola hoop.
Practice tai chi.
Take a yoga class.

When you're wired ...
Do a walking meditation.
Move to music.
Get a massage.

When you're experiencing body boredom...
Take a salsa or swing−dancing class.
Take improvisational acting lessons.
Garden or build sand castles.

When you're stuck in routine...
Take a kick—boxing class.
Go river rafting.
Take a rigorous nature hike.[8]

Mix It Up

Here's a varied selection of movement options.

Every day
Park your car a few blocks away from your destination.
Take the stairs instead of the elevator.
Walk to the store or mailbox.

Three to five times per week
Aerobic exercise:
Walk briskly during your lunch break or after dinner.
Bicycle to and from work or on a stationary bicycle.
Take a dance class.

Recreation:
Practice a martial art such as akido or karate.
Play basketball, softball, or baseball.
Try roller skating in your local park.

Two to three times per week
Flexibility and strength:
Try stretching, yoga, or Pilates.
Do push—ups, curl—ups, and sit—ups.
Lift weights.

Make an "In Motion" Plan

The United States Department of Agriculture (USDA) recommends that adults exercise at least thirty minutes daily; children
and teens should target fifty minutes of activity each day. The
USDA Physical Activity Pyramid offers both moderate and vigorous physical activity possibilities.

Moderate
Walking briskly (about 3½ miles per hour)
Hiking
Gardening
Dancing
Golfing (walking and carrying your own clubs)
Bicycling
Weight training (a general light workout)

Vigorous
Running, jogging (5 miles per hour)
Bicycling (more than 10 miles per hour)
Swimming (freestyle laps)
Aerobics
Walking fast (4½ miles per hour)
Lifting heavy weights
Playing competitive basketball[9]

Get Moving!
Both food and movement have the power to heal in multiple
dimensions—physically, emotionally, spiritually, and socially. Doesn't
movement influence your physical, emotional, spiritual, and social
well-being as well as your weight—in other words, your entire
being? Isn't each facet of physical activity a reflection of the others?
Isn't each both independent and interdependent?

The goal of this chapter has been to give you insights into how
you can expand your vision of what a whole person approach to food,

eating, and achieving your optimal weight can be. We are suggesting that you include whole person exercise options that feed you physi—cally, emotionally, spiritually, and socially—each time you are in action.

Chapter 12

Winning Weight-Loss Strategies

W henever we're teaching or lecturing about optimal eating, based on our whole person nutrition program, we often begin by inviting participants to share their recollections of especially memo— rable meals. Without fail, people include all the *solutions* to the overeating styles. Their stories are filled with food—related pleasure, mindfulness, good feelings, fresh food, and shared dining in a pleasant atmosphere. The meals we hear about are never the seven overeating styles in action: eating fast food, alone, to manage unpleasant feelings, while fretting about high fat content, in a hectic or unpleasant atmosphere.

While thinking about memorable meals, we were riveted to the TV when Mireille Guiliano, the author of *French Women Don't Get Fat*, appeared on *The Oprah Winfrey Show* to tell her story. The French— born CEO of Clicquot, Inc. (Veuve Clicquot's American subsidiary), Guillano had come to the United States as a teenage exchange stu— dent, gained twenty pounds, and then gained ten more when she returned to France and continued her American way of eating.[1]

Guiliano's weight—loss success started with a rock bottom moment when she first returned to France. When she descended from the *SS Rotterdam* in the 1960s, it had been a year since she'd seen her family. Expecting her beret—clad father's face to light up when he saw her, she instead saw him looking stunned. When she came closer, he con— tinued to stare at her. As her brother and American shipmate stood nearby, his first words to his beloved daughter were, *"Tu ressembles à un sac de patates"*—you look like a bag of potatoes.

As hurtful as this was, it wasn't enough to prompt her to take action to lose the twenty pounds she'd gained in the States. Instead, Guiliano continued her American eating habits while attending university in Paris—and gained ten more pounds by Christmas. Then during her holiday break, at the urging of Guiliano's mother, the kind and gentlemanly family physician Dr. Meyer intervened. Losing the weight would be easy, he assured her, once she returned to the French way of eating.

After Guiliano kept a three−week record of what, how much, when, and where she ate, she realized she'd adopted quite a few typically American eating styles. For instance, she ate while walking or standing (task snacking) and grabbed whatever was convenient and available (fast foodism). Permanent change, she realized with the help of the man she now refers to as "Dr. Miracle," called for achieving equilibrium not just in her food choices, but in all aspects of her life. To do this, *she would have to engage her mind.*

During the next three months, Guiliano relearned the way of the French woman. And the weight came off. Guiliano is now in her sixties, and the weight has stayed off—without dieting and excessive exercise. Her secret? She reconnected to her country's fresh−food culinary roots and its pleasurable approach to food, eating, and the aesthetics of dining. When we looked closely at Guiliano's comments to Oprah, it was clear that she did it by overcoming the eating styles linked with overeating: food fretting, task snacking, emotional eating, fast foodism, solo dining, unpleasant atmosphere, and sensory disregard. She mentioned enjoying food and relating to it as a pleasure; eating chocolate or other sweets, but in small portions; not counting calories; not working on her computer when it's time for lunch; snacking on fresh, whole food; eating with friends; eating with her senses and paying attention to the food before her; and finally, perceiving that what, how, where, and with whom she eats is a life−style philosophy.

In Chapter 6, we told you about experiments that imply a mystery as to how we metabolize food. We quoted physician Deepak Chopra on the consciousness we bring to meals: "When you look at nutrition from a purely scientific point of view, there is no place for consciousness. And yet, consciousness could be one of the crucial determinants of the metabolism of food itself." Chopra's comment addresses the power of both measurable nutrients in fresh food and harder–to–measure nutrients that seem to protect our weight and well–being when we eat filled with pleasure, mindfulness, positive feelings, social support, aesthetic awareness, and sensory delight— the ingredients that make up the solutions to the overeating styles. Guiliano might describe this as having to engage her mind in order to be successful at losing weight. Chopra's statement resonates with us because, at its core, it encompasses each of the biological, psycho– logical, spiritual, and social elements of whole person nutrition that are pivotal to true nourishment and making weight loss last.

We're asking you to consider Chopra's insight because the anti– dotes to the seven overeating styles (and chemical cuisine, inadequate sleep, and underexercising) ask that you focus your attention on much more than calorie–counting, weight–watching, fat grams, and carb content. Rather, both the intentional and the unintentional aware– ness you bring to meals impacts the way your mind and body use nutrients and calories. Call it awareness, realization, or perception, the "consciousness" to which Chopra alludes suggests a special sen– sibility or sensitivity—an invisible, hard–to–measure mystery—that somehow plays an essential role in the metabolism of food. When this consciousness is activated, it holds the power to end emotional eating, turn dietary deprivation into dietary delight, neutralize poten– tially artery–clogging cholesterol and fat—and help Frenchwoman Mireille Guiliano stay slim for life.

What is it about overcoming the overeating styles that brings so many benefits? Some time ago, an acquaintance gave us a key to the answer. "My brother married a Frenchwoman, and he, his wife, and their two small children live on the outskirts of Paris," he told us. "When I visited my six–year–old nephew at school, I noticed that he and his classmates were served a warm, full–course lunch on glass plates, which they ate while sitting around a small table, chatting with each other."

We thought about this conversation when our research on whole person nutrition uncovered the seven overeating styles, and again while writing this book about the solutions. Wasn't our friend describing some of the elements of the solutions we've been discussing? Our weight–loss message really comes down to this: eat flavor–filled fresh food, be aware of dining accoutrements, dine with others, savor every bite, and relax. Each time you eat, embrace food as if you were following the antidotes to the overeating styles. And eat this way from childhood through adulthood—for life.[2]

Elemental Overview

The ultimate antidote to weight gain and related ailments is to live all the antidotes to the seven overeating styles each day, and to avoid chemical cuisine, get adequate sleep, and engage in more physical activity. For many, this calls for a changed relationship to food and eating—biologically (eat fresh whole foods and don't diet), emotionally (eat for pleasure), spiritually (eat mindfully, with gratitude and aesthetic awareness), and socially (dine in company).

As you no doubt realize by now, our Rx to the overeating styles reframes optimal nourishment as an eating practice for the whole person—and for a lifetime. However, simply reading about the solutions won't change what and how you eat, nor will it open the door to receiving multidimensional nourishment and achieving your optimal weight. That calls for implementing the antidotes on a daily basis. It's not theory, it's not wishful thinking; it's about being proactive—taking action and making a commitment to changing your relationship to food.

Carefully look over the solutions to the seven overeating styles, as listed in the sidebar. Familiarize yourself with all of them. Having an intimate understanding of each one is pivotal to overcoming overeating, overweight, and obesity. Each time you eat or participate in any food–related activity, remember that all seven elements count, and that optimal nourishment includes both the familiar nutrients in food and the psychological, spiritual, and social nutrients that are missing from the food charts.

Rx: Antidotes to the Seven Overeating Styles

Here are the essential antidotes to each of the seven overeating styles we've discussed in this book.

Food Fretting Rx: Perceive food and the experience of eating as a social, ceremonial, sensual pleasure.

Task Snacking Rx: Bring moment–to–moment nonjudgmental awareness to each aspect of the meal.

Emotional Eating Rx: Eat for pleasure—when you have an appetite and you're experiencing feel–good emotions.

Fast Foodism Rx: Choose fresh, whole food in its natural state as often as possible.

Solo Dining Rx: Share food–related experiences with others.

Unappetizing Atmosphere Rx: Dine in psychologically and aesthetically pleasing surroundings.

Sensory Disregard Rx: Feed your senses when you eat by savoring flavors, aromas, colors, presentation, textures, even sounds.

Overcoming Obstacles

We created the ten solutions in *Make Weight Loss Last* to make it easy for you to practice them daily. Only by actually doing them each day will you be empowered to nourish your physical health, your emotions, your senses, and your social well–being. Be patient with yourself: making such sweeping changes in what, how, where, and even with whom you eat is a process. Changing your relationship to food in order to stay slim for life isn't likely to happen overnight: success takes ongoing nurturing, care, and regard . . . for yourself.

To enhance your chances of success, the following section gives you strategies for overcoming obstacles that may be keeping you from integrating the overeating solutions into your life.

Identifying Your Obstacles

At the beginning of this book, you filled out the "What's Your Eating Style?" profile. Needless to say, every person's profile is different. So, too, are the areas—and degrees—of resistance that you may experience in implementing the solutions and getting the results you want. In the profile, you identified the elements that are challenging for you; others you already do easily. Look over the eating styles you pinpointed as integral aspects of your food life, and therefore the hardest to overcome. Look for these in the following section to discover strategies for moving closer to your biological, psychological, spiritual, and social nutrition goals.

Food Fretting

Obstacle: You perceive the experience of eating as a social, ceremonial, and sensual pleasure, but you continue to be overly concerned about food, calories, and diets.

Strategy: Because so many of us have been taught that it's normal to fret about food and obsess about calories, weight, and dieting, this eating style can be particularly challenging to turn around. But it *is* possible—if you decide to go against the dieting and deprivation norm and, instead, change your relationship to food and eating at its core.

This calls for nothing less than turning diet–think into pleasure–think, every time you eat. Each time you find yourself heading back onto the calorie–counting roller coaster, halt the thought by closing your eyes, inhaling deeply, and then exhaling as you release the thought and the related tension surrounding it. Now, think of food and eating as one of life's greatest gifts . . . and pleasures.

Task Snacking

Obstacle: Though you bring moment–to–moment nonjudgmental awareness to each aspect of a meal, you find it difficult to stay focused.

Strategy: It's natural for thoughts to wander. That's why mindfulness meditation is called a *practice*: it's something you can practice for a lifetime. Here are three steps for bringing mindfulness to all food−related activities—from planning your meal to eating it and then washing dishes afterward.

First, decide to focus on food and eating (or shopping or prepping, and so on); simply become aware that you intend to do this. Second, if you find your attention wandering, gently let go of the thoughts or actions that are interfering with your intention and refocus on food. Finally, hold your intention and commitment to mindfulness and focus your attention back on the food or food−related activity.

Emotional Eating

Obstacle: You eat only for pleasure when you have feel−good feel−ings, but then your food cravings and negative emotions take over, making checking in difficult.
Strategy: Accessing the potent power that food has on your feel−ings—and vice versa—isn't always easy. In fact, our research on the seven eating styles showed us that emotions are more strongly related to overeating than is any other element of the eating styles. The anti−dote: tease out the emotions that are manifest before, during, and after you eat.

This requires a subtle refocusing of attention—a shift of mind and heart, a new way of communicating with yourself and your food. Set aside a specific time prior to eating to observe and acknowledge your feelings without judgment or any impulse to act upon them. Simply *be* with your feelings—even if they're negative ones, even if it's uncomfortable for you.

Fast Foodism

Obstacle: You choose fresh whole food in its natural state as often as possible, but sometimes the carrot cake is more tempting than the carrot.
Strategy: Keep in mind that the optimal food guideline isn't about rigid dietary dogma, or rules and regulations; that's why we've quali−fied this guideline with the phrase "as often as possible." Our intention is to help you think of varied fresh, whole food as your most−of−the−time way of eating, not as yet another diet to follow for a while

before returning to your usual way of eating. If you've accomplished this, congratulate yourself—and enjoy non–whole food if you choose it intentionally and it's no longer typical for you. On the other hand, if you want something sweet but want to keep it fresh and whole, consider dates, figs, or a homemade fruit smoothie.

Solo Dining

Obstacle: You share food–related experiences with others sometimes, but you eat alone more often than not.

Strategy: If you often dine by yourself, the easiest way to change that is to bring others to your table through memory and by reflecting on past meals shared with people you like. As you eat and think of these prior dining experiences, consider what made the meals so memorable. Was it the people? The food? The atmosphere? The conversation? A special holiday or celebration? An outdoor picnic or an impromptu indoor meal? Once you've identified the delightful elements of the shared meal, create a comparable dining event with friends, family members, or coworkers. Take pictures of the occasion and then place the photos of food and friends on your dining table so that you can replicate the experience each time you eat.

Unappetizing Atmosphere

Obstacle: You'd like to dine in psychologically and aesthetically pleasing surroundings, but you don't know where to begin.

Strategy: Both the psychological and the aesthetic surroundings in which you dine influence the meal in many ways. If you typically eat in an atmosphere fraught with fighting, hostility, or loud noises, the most obvious action you can take is to change where you eat—or stop dining with people who create an unpleasant atmosphere. If this isn't an option, ask others if they can put their hostilities on hold while eating.

Aesthetically, small changes can make a big difference: light some candles, play some favorite soothing music, and use your best china. Make the atmosphere as pleasant as you can.

Sensory Disregard

Obstacle: You savor the flavors when you eat, but you're finding it hard to make a meaningful connection to your meals.
Strategy: Receiving meals "through your senses," with an aware—ness of the life—giving mystery in food, is one of the most impor—tant secrets to optimal eating. Regard and acknowledge all aspects of the meal before you—from nature as its creator to the farmer who raised the crops. Identify at least one aspect of food to appreciate (for instance, nature and the elements of rain, earth, air, and sunshine).

Perceive food (both plant— and animal—based) as an equal, in that it contains the mystery of life just as we humans do. As you eat, con—sider the alchemy, the interconnection, the oneness inherent in food and eating. Holding appreciation in your heart, focus on the food's flavors. Make a brief blessing of appreciation: thank you for being.

More Strategies

There are additional steps you can take to break through obstacles that keep you from getting and staying on track to make weight loss last. For instance, you can take a quick refresher course by rereading the chapters on the eating issues that are keeping you from being successful. Then review the abundance of solutions presented within the chapters.

Empower yourself to overcome existing obstacles by doing this mini—exercise:

1. Identify the eating style or element—`, sleep, or physical activity—that's most challenging for you personally.

2. Write it down.

3. Identify the reasons you think this is hardest for you.

4. Create your own techniques for overcoming the obstacle(s) you've pinpointed. You can do this by finding the solutions in the chapters that strike the strongest chord with you.

5. Ask yourself this: for the elements you *don't* resist or find challenging, why do you think this is so? Apply these insights to the elements you do find challenging.

Moonlight Memory

"I'm thinking of charging everyone extra for the full moon and moonlight," announced chef Ruggero Gigli in his thick Italian accent from the outdoor porch of Villa Gigli, the combination restaurant and artist studio in Markleeville, California, that's owned by Gigli and his wife, Gina.

A native of Florence, Gigli made the announcement to a hundred or so diners eating and conversing at long tables in his restaurant's garden. He called our attention to the resplendent moonlit setting just as we were about to embark on the first course of our meal: an exquisitely colored and perfectly flavored, textured, and scented pumpkin soup (*zuppa di zucca*). At Villa Gigli, a first course is more, much more than a simple soup or starter: it is all the solutions to the seven overeating styles—food fretting, task snacking, emotional eating, fast foodism, solo dining, unappetizing atmosphere, and sensory disregard—put into action.

As we dined at Villa Gigli that magical evening, we couldn't help but realize how every aspect of the meal embodied the solutions to the overeating styles. We delighted in the entire experience. We focused on the food as we ate, filled with joy and gratitude. The food was exquisitely fresh. Without distraction, we relished every aspect of the evening; we were dining with others in extraordinary surroundings, and we took the time to truly taste and savor our food.

A Taste for All Reasons

In *Make Weight Loss Last*, we've shown you how to eat optimally by explaining and demystifying seven overeating styles—and the nutritional dimensions that don't show up on food charts. This new/

ancient view asks that you pay attention to all of the eating styles each time you eat—and practice their antidotes every day.

The ultimate message is simple: the healing gifts of food are available each time you eat. As a matter of fact, every time you shop for, prepare, and eat food, you have the opportunity make weight loss last. Along the way, you're empowering yourself to experience food as the symphonic sensory masterpiece that it is—with notes of fresh food, positive feelings, in−the−moment mindfulness, culinary delight, pleasing surroundings, rich flavors, and social interaction.

Weaving together the moments of a meal based on these ele− ments means you're consciously connecting to what you're eating, how you're eating, and with whom you're eating. This isn't an easy task, for in our hurry−worry society, most of us no longer enjoy meals of fresh, whole food at the dining room table, filled with a sense of quietude, with people we love—unless we're living the ele− ments of optimal eating discussed throughout this book. When you eat from such a place of pleasure, you're fed more than food. Each dining experience becomes an occasion to nourish your entire being, and to turn the tide of weight gain.

Taking pleasure in food, eating mindfully, nourishing yourself with positive emotions as you eat, savoring flavors and surround− ings, eating with others, quitting chemical cuisine, getting restor− ative sleep, and integrating movement into your life—these are at the heart of achieving and maintaining optimal weight and well−being. Remember that it is a process, a lifetime adventure you can take to nourish your biological, psychological, spiritual, and social well− being each time you eat, sleep, and get moving.

The ten solutions in *Make Weight Loss Last* are a template not only for what and how to eat, but also for how to live: consciously, filled with the sense of wonder inherent in the alchemical union of human beings, food, weight, sleep, and physical activity. The solutions we've told you about throughout this book are resplendent with possibili− ties for nourishing every aspect of your being, every day . . . for life.

References, Notes, and Links

Preface to the New Edition

1. Deborah Kesten and Larry Scherwitz, *The Enlightened Diet: 7 Weight-Loss Solutions That Nourish Body, Mind, and Soul* (Berkeley, CA: Ten Speed Press, 2007).

2. Larry Scherwitz and Deborah Kesten, "Seven Eating Styles Linked to Overeating, Overweight, and Obesity," *Explore: The Journal of Science and Healing* 1, no. 5 (2005): 342–59.

3. The seven eating styles are based on the authors' research for their first book, *Feeding the Body, Nourishing the Soul* (Berkeley, CA: Conari Press, 1997; Amherst, MA: White River Press, 2007).

4. Deborah Kesten, *The Healing Secrets of Food: A Practical Guide for Nourishing Body, Mind, and Soul* (Novato, CA: New World Library, 2001).

Introduction
Make Weight Loss Last: The 10 Solutions

1. Gayle King, *CBS This Morning*, CBS–TV, New York, April 1, 2012.

2. Y. C. Wang, K. McPherson, T. Marsh et al., "Health and Economic Burden of the Projected Obesity Trends in the USA and the UK," *The Lancet* 378, no. 9793 (2011): 815–25.

3. C. Ogden, M. Carroll, L. Curtin et al., "Prevalence of High Body Mass Index in US Children and Adolescents, 2007–2008," *Journal of the American Medical Association* 303, no. 3 (2010): 242

4. National Center for Health Statistics. Health, United States, with Special Features on Death and Dying. Hyattsville, MD; U.S. Department of Health and Human Services, 2011.

5. B. Moss and W. Yeaton,"Young Children's Weight Trajectories and Associated Risk Factors: Results from the Early Childhood Longitudinal Study–Birth Cohort," *American Journal of Health Promotion* 25, no. 3 (2011): 190–8.

6. Taylor Hibma, "5 Causes of Obesity in America," eHow.com, www.ehow.com/how–does_5558417_causes–obesity–america. html#ixzz1pE8z6X51 (accessed March 18, 2012).

7. A. Gearhardt, S. Yokum, P. Orr et al.,"Neural Correlates of Food Addiction," *Archives of General Psychiatry* 68, no. 8 (2011): 808–16.

8. D. Ornish, L. W. Scherwitz, R. S. Doody et al.,"Effects of Stress Management Training and Dietary Changes in Treating Ischemic Heart Disease," *Journal of the American Medical Association* 249, no. 1 (1983): 54–9.

9. L. Scherwitz, D. Kesten, O. Brusis et al., "Are Comprehensive Lifestyle Changes Possible in German Heart Patients?" Pilot study findings. *Progression and Regression of Atherosclerosis*, W. Koenig, V. Hombach, M. Bond, D. Kramsch, editors (Vienna: Blackwell–MZV, 1995).

10. S. Olshansky, D. Passaro, R. Hershow et al.,"A Potential Decline in Life Expectancy in the United States in the 21st Century," *New England Journal of Medicine* 352, no. 11 (2005): 1138–45.

11. D. Ornish, S. Brown, L. Scherwitz et al.,"Can Lifestyle Changes Reverse Coronary Heart Disease? The Lifestyle Heart Trial," *Lancet* 336, no. 8708 (1990): 129–33.

12. L. Scherwitz et al., "Are Comprehensive Lifestyle Changes Possible in German Heart Patients?"

13. Deborah Kesten, *Feeding the Body, Nourishing the Soul* (Berkeley, CA: Conari Press, 1997; Amherst, MA: White River Press, 2007).

14. Deborah Kesten, "The Enlightened Diet: Integrating Biological, Spiritual, Social, and Psychological Nutrition," *Spirituality & Health* 4 (Winter 2003): 29–39

15. Deborah Kesten, "The Enlightened Diet Integrative Eating E–course," *Spirituality & Health* (December 16, 2002–January 24, 2003). Available at www.EnlightenedDiet.com.

16. The implications of our study are enormous, because not only did we discover seven new overeating styles strongly linked with being over–weight and obese, we learned that those who made the most changes in the overeating styles during the study lost the most weight. In other words, the more people improved across all seven overeating styles over the eighteen–week e–course, the more likely they were to lose weight. Perhaps even more inspirational is the realization that they were able to make dramatic changes in their overeating styles on their own.

17. Another contribution of the overeating styles is that they offer a "whole person" perspective on why so many of us gain weight and struggle with taking and keeping it off. They provide us with direction for over–coming the various reasons we overeat in order to make weight loss last. For weight–loss success, identify your problem eating style and then remedy the key problem behavior that is the root cause of your weight gain.

18. Kelly Brownell, Open Yale Courses, Psyc 123: The Psychology, Biology and Politics of Food, Lecture 2, "Food Then, Food Now: Modern Food Conditions and Their Mismatch with Evoluton." www.oyc.yale.edu/psychology/psyc–123 (accessed March 8, 2012).

Chapter 1: What's Your Overeating Style?

1. Larry Scherwitz and Deborah Kesten, "Seven Eating Styles Linked to Overeating, Overweight, and Obesity," *Explore: The Journal of Science and Healing* 1, no. 5 (2005): 342–59.

2. Deborah Kesten, *The Healing Secrets of Food: A Practical Guide for Nourishing Body, Mind, and Soul* (Novato, CA: New World Library, 2001): 3–18.

3. Deborah Kesten, "The Enlightened Diet: Integrating Biological, Spiritual, Social, and Psychological Nutrition," *Spirituality & Health* 4 (Winter 2003): 29–39.

Chapter 2: Jettison Judgment

1. K. M. Flegal, M. D. Carroll, R. J. Kuczmarski, and C. L. Johnson, "Overweight and Obesity in the United States: Prevalence and Trends," *International Journal of Obesity* 22 (1998): 39–47; A. H. Mokdad, M. K. Serdula, W. H. Dietz et al., "The Spread of the Obesity Epidemic in the United States," *Journal of the American Medical Association* 282, no. 16 (1999): 1519–22.

2. C. Ogden, M. Carroll, L. Curtin et al., "Prevalence of High Body Mass Index in US Children and Adolescents, 2007–2008," *Journal of the American Medical Association* 303, no. 3 (2010): 242–9.

3. G. D. Foster and T. A. Wadden, "What Is a Reasonable Weight Loss? Patients' Expectations and Evaluations of Obesity Treatment Outcomes," *Journal of Consulting and Clinical Psychology* 65, no. 1 (1997): 79–85; G. D. Foster, T. A. Wadden, S. Phelan, D. B. Sarwer et al., "Obese Patients' Perceptions of Treatment Outcomes and the Factors That Influence Them," *Archives of Internal Medicine* 161, no. 17 (2001): 2133–39.

4. R. Dalle Grave, S. Calugi, E. Molinari, M. L. Petroni et al., "Weight Loss Expectations in Obese Patients and Treatment Attrition: An Observational Multicenter Study," *Obesity Research* 1311 (November 2005): 1961–69.

5. Tufts University, "Yes, but Is Weight Loss the Be–all and the End–all?" *Tufts Health & Nutrition Letter*, July 2004, www.healthletter.tufts.edu/issues/2004–07/ weight.html (accessed June 15, 2007); Christopher D. Still, "Health Benefits of Modest Weight Loss—Penn State Geisinger Health Care System," *Healthology, Inc.*, 2006, www.weightfocus.com (accessed March 16, 2006).

6. M. L. Dansinger, J. A. Gleason, J. L. Griffith et al., "Comparison of the Atkins, Ornish, Weight Watchers, and Zone Diets for Weight Loss and Heart Disease Risk Reduction: A Randomized Trial," *Journal of the American Medical Association* 293, no. 1 (2005): 43–53; Daniel DeNoon, "4 Diets Face Off: Which Is the Winner? The Best Diet: The One You Stick With," *WebMd Medical News*, January 4, 2005, www.webmd.com (accessed July 24, 2006).

7. C. C. DiClemente and J. O. Prochaska, "Self Change and Therapy Change of Smoking Behavior: A Comparison of Processes of Change in Cessation and Maintenance," *Addictive Behaviors* 89 (1982): 133–42; J. O. Prochaska and C. C. DiClemente, "Trans–theoretical Therapy: Toward a More Integrative Model of Change," *Psychotherapy: Theory, Research and Practice* 19 (1982): 276–88.

8. Psychology Matters, APA Online, "Understanding How People Change Is First Step in Changing Unhealthy Behavior," www.psychologymatters.org/dicle–mente (accessed December 21, 2006); Robert Westermeyer, "A User–Friendly Model of Change," Habit Smart, September 5, 2005, www.habitsmart.com/ motivate.htm (accessed December 21, 2006).

9. *The American Heritage Dictionary of the English Language*, 4th ed., s.v. "diet."

Chapter 3: Focus on Food

1. Healthwatch, "Car Cuisine: Food Industry Caters to Drivers Eating Behind the Wheel," *CBS News*, November 9, 2005, www.cbsnews.com/ stories/2005/11/09/health/ main1029857.shtml (accessed October 11, 2006).

2. Nanci Hellmich and Jo dee Black, "Desktop dining: recipe for disaster," *Great Falls Tribune,* March 1, 2004, www.greatfallstribune.com/news/stories/20040301/localnews/49568.html (accessed August 2006).

3. Donald R. Morse and M. L. Furst, "Meditation: An In–depth Study," *Journal of the American Society of Psychosomatic Dentistry and Medicine* 29, no. 5 (1982): 1–96.

4. Herbert Benson, *The Relaxation Response* (New York: William Morrow, 1975).

5. Deborah Kesten, *Feeding the Body, Nourishing the Soul: Essentials of Eating for Physical, Emotional, and Spiritual Well-Being* (Berkeley, CA: Conari Press, 1997; Amherst, MA: White River Press, 2007).

6. Urasenke Foundation, "The Urasenke Tradition of Chado" (Kyoto, Japan: Urasenke Foundation, 1995).

7. G. D. Jacobs, "The Physiology of Mind–Body Interactions: The Stress Response and the Relaxation Response," *Journal of Alternative and Complementary Medicine* 8, no. 2 (2002): supplement 1: 58392.

8. R. J. Davidson, "Alterations in Brain and Immune Function Produced by Mindfulness Meditation," *Psychosomatic Medicine* 66, no. 1 (2004): 147–52.

9. Jean Kristeller, "An Exploratory Study of a Meditation–Based Intervention for Binge Eating Disorder," *Journal of Health Psychology* 4, no. 3 (1999): 357–63.

10. Jean Kristeller, "Know Your Hunger," *Spirituality & Health* 8, no. 2 (2005).

11. J. J. Daubenmier, G. Weidner, M. Sumner, N. Mendell et al., "The Contribution of Changes in Diet, Exercise, and Stress Management to Changes in Coronary Risk in Women and Men in the Multisite Cardiac Lifestyle Intervention Program," *Annals of Behavioral Medicine* 33 (January 2007).

12. Gerdi Weidner (PhD, vice president and director of research, Preventive Medicine Research Institute, Sausalito, CA), conversation with Deborah Kesten, October 20, 2006.

13. Ibid.

Chapter 4: Access Your Appetite

1. Barbara Birsinger (PhD in theology, registered dietitian), conversation with Deborah Kesten during the week of September 26, 2006.

2. Cassandra Vieten (PhD, clinical psychologist and research scientist, San Francisco and Petaluma, CA), conversation with Deborah Kesten, February 8, 2005.

3. Judith J. Wurtman, *Managing Your Mind and Mood through Food* (New York: Rawson Associates, 1986).

4. Eckhart Tolle, *The Power of Now* (Novato, CA: New World Library, 1999).

5. Vieten, February 8, 2005.

6. Overeaters Anonymous, www.oa.org/lifeline_monthly.html (accessed December 8, 2006).

7. Birsinger, September 26, 2006.

8. Barbara Birsinger, "Abstract: Effects of an Integrative Approach on Restoring Balance to Eating and Weight Issues" (Holos University Graduate Seminary, February 2006).

9. Instruments used by Barbara Birsinger for pre– and post–intervention tests:

   (1) Intuitive Eating Scale (IES), 26 items: measures intrinsic eating, extrinsic eating, antidieting behaviors, and self–care practices. Hala Madanat, Jaylyn Hawks, and Ashley Harris, "The Intuitive Eating Scale:

Development and Preliminary Validation," *American Journal of Health Education* 35, no. 2 (2004): 90.

(2) Motivation for Eating Scale (MES), 43 items: measures emotional, physical, and environmental subscales in relation to motivation for eating. Steven Hawks, Cari Merrill, Julie Gast, and Jaylyn Hawks, *Ecology of Food and Nutrition* 43 (2004): 307–26.

(3) Dutch Eating Behavior Questionnaire (DEBQ), 33 items: measures restrained, emotional, and external eating behaviors. T. van Strien, J. E. R. Fritjers, G. P. A. Bergers, and P. B. Defares, "The Dutch Eating Behavior Questionnaire for Assessment of Restrained, Emotional, and External Eating Behavior," *International Journal of Eating Disorders* 5 (1986): 295–315.

(4) Eating Attitudes Test (EAT), 26 items: screening measure for eating pathology. D. Garner et al., "Eating Attitudes Test," *Psychological Medicine* 12, no. 4 (1982): 71–78.

(5) Spiritual Well–Being Scale (SWBS), 20 items: measures subscales of existential and religious spiritual well–being. Craig W. Ellison, "Toward an Integrative Measure of Health and Well–Being," *Journal of Psychology and Theology* 19, no. 1 (1991): 35–48.

(6) Rosenberg Self–Esteem Scale (RSES), 10 items: measures general feelings of self–esteem. M. Rosenberg, *Society and the Adolescent Self-Image* (Middletown, CT: Wesleyan University Press, 1965).

(7) Body Satisfaction Scale (BSS), 21 items: measures satisfaction with one's physical appearance. E. Stice, "A Prospective Test of the Dual Pathway Model of Bulimic Pathology: Mediating Effects of Dieting and Negative Affect," *Journal of Abnormal Psychology* 110 (2001): 124–35.

(8) Bem Sex Role Inventory (BSRI), 60 items: measures masculine/ feminine orientation. S. L. Bem, "The Measurement of Psychological Androgeny," *Journal of Clinical and Consulting Psychology* 42 (1974): 155–62.

(9) Body Mass Index (BMI): measures height and weight relationship to assess whether a person is overweight or obese.

(10) Food Habits Questionnaire: developed by Barbara Birsinger to measure qualitative dietary intake.

10. Barbara Birsinger, "Conversations with Body: Discovering the Spiritual Archetypal and Symbolic Messages in Food, Eating, Body Language, and Weight" workshop, "Weekly Topics—Intended Results, Methods, and Measures," 2005.

11. Judith Wurtman, *Managing Your Mind and Mood through Food* (New York: Perennial/HarperCollins, 1988).

Chapter 5: Get Fresh

1. Mark Hyman, "Systems Biology: The Gut–Brain–Fat Cell Connection and Obesity," *Alternative Therapies* 12, no. 1 (2006): 10.

2. Judith C. Rodriguez, "Fast Foods Health," *Gale Encyclopedia of Nutrition and Well Being* (New York: Gale Group, 2004), www.healthline.com/galecontent/fast-foods (accessed June 15, 2007).

3. James J. Ferguson, "Definition of Terms Used in the National Organic Program" (Gainesville: University of Florida, Institute of Food and Agricultural Sciences, Horticultural Sciences Department, Florida Cooperative Extension Service, January 2004), www.edis.ifas.ufl.edu/HS209 (accessed May 1, 2007).

4. Yourdictionary.com (accessed June 11, 2007), s.v. "junk food."

5. William Saletan, "It's a Fat, Fat, Fat, Fat World," *San Francisco Chronicle*, September 17, 2006, E3; David Goldstein, "Junk–Food Makers Face FTC Scrutiny," *San Francisco Chronicle*, November 18, 2006, A8; Kim Severson, "Sugar Coated: We're Drowning in High Fructose Corn Syrup," *San Francisco Chronicle*, February 18, 2004, E6.

6. Bridget Murray, "Fast−Food Culture Serves Up Super−Size Americans," *Monitor on Psychology* 32, no. 11 (2001), www.apa.org/monitor/dec01/fastfood.html (accessed June 15, 2007).

7. Robert H. Lustig, "Childhood Obesity: Behavioral Aberration or Biochemical Drive? Reinterpreting the First Law of Thermodynamics," *Nature Clinical Practice Endocrinology & Metabolism* 8 (2006): 447–58.

8. "McDonald's USA Ingredients Listing for Popular Menu Items," http://nutri−tion.mcdonalds.com/getnutrition/ingredientslist.pdf (accessed January 13, 2007).

9. "Sugar: Sweet by Nature," advertisement, *News Tribune* (Tacoma, WA), December 7, 2006.

10. Michael F. Roizen and Mehmet C. Oz, "Food Fight: The Ghrelin versus Leptin Grudge Match," *You: On a Diet* (New York: Free Press, 2006).

11. Michael Thomas Lueck and Kim Severson, "New York Bans Most Trans Fats in Restaurants," *New York Times*, December 6, 2006, www.nytimes.com/2006/12/06nyrefgion/06fat.html (accessed December 6, 2006); Georgia Jones, "Fast Foods! A 4−H Lifelong Learning Resource," *Journal of Nutrition Education and Behavior* 38, no. 4 (2006): supple−ment S37; Bonnie Liebman, "The Pressure to Eat," *Nutrition Action* (July/August 1998), www.cspinet.org/nah/7_98eat.htm (accessed June 15, 2007); "Fast Food," Wikipedia, www.en.wikipedia.org/wiki/Fast_food (accessed December 5, 2006); D. Mozaffarian, M. B. Katan, A. Ascherio, M. Stampfer, and W. C. Willett, "Trans Fatty Acids and Cardiovascular Disease," *New England Journal of Medicine* 354, no. 1 (2006): 1601–13; F. B. Hu, R. M. van Dam, and S. Liu, "Diet and Risk of Type II Diabetes: The Role of Types of Fat and Carbohydrate," *Diabetologia* 44, no. 7 (2001): 805–17; R. M. van Dam, M. Stampfer, W. C. Willett, F. B. Hu, and E. B. Rimm, "Dietary Fat and Meat Intake in Relation to Risk of Type 2 Diabetes in Men," *Diabetes Care* 25, no. 3 (2002): 417–24; Anna Gosline, "Why Fast Foods Are Bad, Even in Moderation," *New Scientist* (June

12, 2006), www.newscientist.com/article.ns?id=dn9318&feed1d=online-news_rss20 (accessed June 15, 2007).

12. Connie Guttersen, "America's Supersized Waistlines," Foodservice: Recent Findings, www.calolive.org/foodservice/findings/ findings_ 2003q1.html (accessed December 2, 2006); Jeanie Lerche Davis, "Fast Food Creates Fat Kids," *WebMD Medical News* (January 5, 2004), www.webmd.com/content/ article/79/96083.htm (accessed December 6, 2006); Robert H. Lustig, "Childhood Obesity," 447–58; "WHO–MONICA Project: Risk Factors," abstract, *International Journal of Epidemiology* 18 (1989), supplement 1: S46–55.

13. G. Ma, Y. Li, Y. Wu, F. Zhai, Z. Cui, X. Hu, et al., "The Prevalence of Body Overweight and Obesity and Its Changes among Chinese People during 1992 to 2002," *Chinese Journal of Preventive Medicine* 39 (2005): 311–15 (in Chinese, with English abstract); Y. Wu, G. Ma, Y. Hu, Y. Li, X. Li, Z. Cui et al., "The Current Prevalence Status of Body Overweight and Obesity in China: Data from the China Nutrition and Health Survey," *Chinese Journal of Preventive Medicine* 39 (2005): 316–20 (in Chinese, with English abstract).

14. Dean Ornish, *Eat More, Weigh Less: Dr. Dean Ornish's Life Choice Program for Losing Weight Safely while Eating Abundantly* (New York: HarperCollins, 1993).

15. Julie Meyer, "10 Best Slimming Foods," *Woman's Day* (October 3, 2006), 96.

Chapter 6: Enjoy Food with Others

1. The National Center on Addiction and Substance Abuse (CASA) at Columbia University, www.casacolumbia.org (accessed November 9, 2007).

2. M. W. Gillman, S. L. Rifas–Shiman, A.L. Frazier, et al, "Family Dinner and Diet Quality among Older Children and Adolescents," *Archives of Family Medicine* 9 (March 2000): 235–40.

3. Richard S. Strauss and Harold A. Pollack, "Epidemic Increase in Childhood Overweight, 1986–1998," *Journal of the American Medical Association* 286, no. 22 (2001): 2845–48.

4. Julie Stewart Wolf and John G. Bruhn, *The Power of Clan: The Influence of Human Relationships on Heart Disease* (New Brunswick, NJ: Transaction, 1993).

5. Robert M. Nerem, Murina J. Levesque, and J. Fredrick Cornhill, "Social Environment as a Factor in Diet–Induced Atherosclerosis," *Science New Series* 208, no. 4451 (1980): 1475–76.

6. Deepak Chopra, *Body, Mind and Soul*, PBS, KQED–TV, San Francisco, March 7, 1995.

7. Marion Cunningham, conversation with Deborah Kesten, April 2003.

8. Vinita Azarow, conversation with Deborah Kesten.

9. "Dream Dinners: Where Wonderful Meals Come True," www.dreamdinners.com (accessed January 3, 2007).

Chapter 7: Dine by Design

1. Elsie M. Widdowson, "Mental Contentment and Physical Growth," *The Lancet* 1, no. 24 (June 16, 1951): 1316–18.

2. Reginald Horsman, *Frontier Doctor William Beaumont, America's First Great Medical Scientist* (Columbia, MO: University of Missouri Press, 1996).

3. Candace B. Pert, *Molecules of Emotion: Why You Feel the Way You Feel* (New York: Scribner, 1997), 297–98.

4. N. Garg, B. Wansink, and J. Jeffrey, "The Influence of Incidental Affect on Consumers' Food Intake," *Journal of Marketing* 71, no. 1 (2007), 194.

5. Marc Schweitzer et al., "Healing Spaces: Elements of Environmental Design That Make an Impact on Health," *The Journal of Alternative and Complementary Medicine* 10 (2004), supplement 1: S71–S83.

6. L. Scherwitz and D. Kesten, "Seven Eating Styles Linked to Overeating, Overweight, and Obesity," *Explore: The Journal of Science and Healing* 1, no. 5 (2005): 342–59.

7. Christine Aaron in conversation with author Mireille Guiliano and Oprah Winfrey, "Anti–Aging Breakthroughs," transcript, *The Oprah Winfrey Show*, May 17, 2005 (Livingston, NJ: Burrelle's Information Services), 21.

Chapter 8: Feed the Senses

1. Mark Morford, "Obese American Tourists, Ho!" Notes & Errata, *San Francisco Chronicle*, February 22, 2006, www.sfgate.com/ cgi–bin/article.cgi?f=/gate/archive/2006/02/22/notes022206.DTL&nl=fix (accessed June 15, 2007).

2. Seth Roberts, "What Makes Food Fattening? A Pavlovian Theory of Weight Control" (theory article, University of California, Berkeley, February 2005), 1–77.

3. Dennis Prager, "Instant Willpower!" *Woman's World* 27, no. 40 (2006), 18–19.

4. Seth Roberts, *The Shangri-La Diet* (New York: G.P. Putnam's Sons, 2006).

5. Keri Brenner, "Dissecting the Shangri–La Diet Fad," *The Olympian*, July 31, 2006, B8.

6. Hildegard of Bingen, *Secrets of God: Writings of Hildegard of Bingen*, ed. Sabrina FlanShambhala, 1996).

7. Barbara Birsinger, "Conversations with Bod" workshop, "Weekly Topics— Intended Results, Methods, and Measures," 2005.

8. Birsinger, September 26, 2006.

9. Namgyal Qusar, First International Conference on Tibetan Medicine, Washington, D.C., November 7–9, 1998.

10. Michael Mayer (PhD, psychologist, Orinda, CA), conversation with Deborah Kesten, December 5, 1996.

Chapter 9: Quit Chemical Cuisine

1. J. Kim, K. E. Peterson, K. S. Scanlon et al., "Trends in Overweight from 1980 through 2001 among Preschool–Aged Children Enrolled in a Health Maintenance Organization," *Obesity* 14, no. 7 (2006): 1107–12.

2. A.V. Krishnan, P. Stathis, S. F. Permuth et al.,"Bisphenol–A: An Estrogenic Substance Is Released from Polycarbonate Flasks During Autoclaving," *Endocrinology* 132, no. 6 (1993): 2279–86.

3. Breast Cancer Fund, "Chemicals in Plastics," http://www.breastcancerfund. org/clear–science/chemicals–linked–to–breast–cancer/plastics/ (accessed February 6, 2012).

4. I. A. Lang, T. S. Galloway, A. Scarlett et al.,"Association of Urinary Bisphenol a Concentration with Medical Disorders and Laboratory Abnormalities in Adults," *The Journal of the American Medical Association* 300, no. 11 (2008): 1303–10.

5. R. W. Stahlhut, E. van Wijngaarden, T. D. Dye et al.,"Concentrations of Urinary Phthalate Metabolites Are Associated with Increased Waist Circumference and Insulin Resistance in Adult U.S. Males," *Environmental Health Perspectives* 115, no. 6 (2007): 876–82.

6. D. H. LeeI, K. Lee, H. Jin et al.,"Association between Serum Concentrations of Persistent Organic Pollutants and Insulin Resistance among Nondiabetic Adults: Results from the National Health and Nutrition Examination Survey 1999–2002," *Diabetes Care* 30, no. 3 (2007): 622–8.

7. O. Vasiliu, L. Cameron, J. Gardiner et al.,"Polybrominated Biphenyls, Polychlorinated Biphenyls, Body Weight, and Incidence of Adult–Onset Diabetes Mellitus," *Epidemiology* 17, no. 4 (2006): 352–9.

8. H. Masuno, T. Kidani, K. Sekiya et al.,"Bisphenol a in Combination with Insulin Can Accelerate the Conversion of 3T3–L1 Fibroblasts to Adipocytes," *Journal of Lipid Research* 43, no. 5 (2002): 676–84.

9. F. Grün, H. Watanabe, Z. Zamanian et al., "Endocrine–Disrupting Organotin Compounds Are Potent Inducers of Adipogenesis in Vertebrates," *Molecular Endocrinology* 20, no. 9 (2006): 2141–55.

10. T. Colborn, J. Myers, D. Dumanoski, "CHE Partnership Call: Endocrine Disruption and Environmental Health: Ten Years after Our Stolen Future," March 22, 2006, http://www.healthandenvironment.org/articles/partnership calls/346 (accessed February 5, 2012).

11. CBC News, Health, "Years of Exposure to BPA Linked to Health Risks in Humans," September 16, 2008, http://www.cbc.ca/news/health/ story/2008/09/15/bpa–jama.html (accessed February 5, 2012).

12. Leah Zerbe, "BPA to Be Banned by Congress," May 17, 2010, www. rodale.com/bpa–and–health–risks (accessed February 5, 2012).

13. C. A. Dyer, "Heavy Metals as Endocrine Disrupting Chemicals," in A.C. Gore (ed.), *Endocrine Disrupting Chemicals: From Basic Research to Clinical Practice*, pp 111–33 (Totowa, NJ: Humana Press, 2007).

14. Paul Goettlich, "What are Endocrine Disruptors?," August 8, 2006, http://www.mindfully.org/Pesticide/EDs–PWG–16jun01.htm (accessed February 5, 2012).

15. R. J. Kavlock, G. P. Daston, C. DeRosa et al., "Research Needs for the Risk Assessment of Health and Environmental Effects of Endocrine Disruptors: A Report of the U.S. EPA–Sponsored Workshop," *Environtal Health Perspectives* 104, supplement 4 (1996): 715–40.

16. F. S. vom Saal and C. Hughes, "An Extensive New Literature Concerning Low–Dose Effects of Bisphenol A Shows the Need for a New Risk Assessment," *Environmental Health Perspectives* 113, no. 8 (2005): 926–33.

17. F. Grün, B. Blumberg, "Perturbed Nuclear Receptor Signaling by Environmental Obesogens as Emerging Factors in the Obesity Crisis," *Reviews in Endocrine & Metabolic Disorders* 8, no. 2 (2007): 161–71.

18. Beth Daley, "Is Plastic Making Us Fat?", *Boston Globe*, January 14, 2008, http://www.boston.com/news/health/articles/2008/01/14/is_plastic_making_us_fat/ (accessed February 6, 2012).

19. Tom Vasich, "Big on Obesogens," http://www.uci.edu/features/2009/10/feature_ obesogens_091019,php (accessed February 6, 2012).

20. *The Dr. Oz Show*, "Understanding Obesogens," September 20, 2010, www.doctoroz.com/videos/understanding–obesogens (accessed February 5, 2012).

21. Sharon Begley, *The Daily Beast*, from *Newsweek Magazine*, "Born to be Big, Early Exposure to Common Chemicals May be Programming Kids to be Fat," September 10, 2009, http://www.thedailybeast.com/news-week/2009/09/10/born-to-be-big.html (accessed February 4, 2012).

22. T. Takeuchi, O. Tsutsumi, Y. Ikezuki et al.,"Positive Relationship between Androgen and the Endocrine Disruptor, Bisphenol A, in Normal Women and Women with Ovarian Dysfunction," *Endocrine journal* 51, no. 2 (2004): 165–9.

23. D. Melzer, N. Rice, M. H. Depledge et al.,"Association between Serum Perfluorooctanoic Acid (PFOS) and Thyroid Disease in the U.S. National Health and Nutrition Examination Survey," *Environmental Health Perspectives* 118, no. 5 (2010): 686–92.

24. R. R. Newbold, E. Padilla–Banks, R. J. Snyder et al.,"Developmental Exposure to Estrogenic Compounds and Obesity," *Birth Defects Research. Part A, Clinical and Molecular Teratology* 73, no. 7 (2005): 478–80.

25. B. L. Strom, R. Schinnar, E. E. Ziegler et al., "Exposure to Soy–Based Formula in Infancy and Endocrinological and Reproductive Outcomes in Young Adulthood," *Journal of the American Medical Association* 286, no. 7 (2001): 807–14.

26. Begley, "Born to be Big," September 10, 2009.

27. Gray Graham, Deborah Kesten, Larry Scherwitz, *Pottenger's Prophecy: How Food Resets Genes for Wellness or Illness* (Amherst, MA : White River Press, 2011).

28. Carol Ann Sayles , conversation with Deborah Kesten, February 19, 2012; website for Boggy Creek Farm, Austin, Texas: www.boggycreek–farm.com.

29. Jane Houlihan, Environmental Working Group, "PCBs in Farmed Salmon," July 2003, http://www.ewg.org/reports/farmedpcbs (accessed February 4, 2012).

30. Food Marketing Institute, "Natural and Organic Foods: Executive Summary," June 2007, http://www.fmi.org/media/bg/natural_organic_foods.pdf (accessed February 6, 2012).

31. Paul Goettlich, "PVC: A Health Hazard from Production through Disposal," October 25, 2001, http://www.mindfully.org/Plastic/Polyvinylchloride/PVC–Health–HazardPWG25oct01.htm (accessed February 6, 2012).

32. S. Kirchner, T. Kieu, C. Chow et al.,"Prenatal Exposure to the Environmental Obesogen Tributyltin Predisposes Multipotent Stem Cells to Become Adipocytes," *Molecular Endocrinology* 24, no. 3 (2010): 526–39.

33. E. P. Hines, S. S. White, J. P. Stanko et al.,"Phenotypic Dichotomy following Developmental Exposure to Perfluorooctanoic Acid (PFOA) in Female CD–1 Mice: Low Doses Induce Elevated Serum Leptin

and Insulin, and Overweight in Mid–Life," *Molecular and Cellular Endocrinology"* 304, no. 1–2 (2009): 97–105.

Chapter 10: Sleep More, Weigh Less

1. S. R. Patel, A. Malhotra, D. P. White et al., "Association between Reduced Sleep and Weight Gain in Women," *American Journal of Epidemiology* 164, no. 10 (2006): 947–54.

2. G. Hasler, D. J. Buysse, R. Klaghofer et al.,"The Association between Short Sleep Duration and Obesity in Young Adults: A 13–Year Prospective Study," *Sleep* 27, no. 4 (2004): 661–6.

3. F. P. Cappuccio, F. M. Taggart, N. B. Kandala et al.,"Meta–Analysis of Short Sleep Duration and Obesity in Children and Adults," *Sleep* 31, no. 5 (2008): 619–26.

4. S. Taheri, "The Link between Short Sleep Duration and Obesity: We Should Recommend More Sleep to Prevent Obesity," *Archives of Disease in Childhood* 91, no. 11 (2006): 881–4.

5. U.S. Department of Health and Human Services: National Institutes of Health, National Heart, Lung, and Blood Institute, "Your Guide to Healthy Sleep," NIH Publication No. 06–5271, November 2005, http://www.nhlbi.nih.gov/health/public/sleep/yg_slp.htm (accessed February 16, 2012).

6. G. Jacobs, The National Sleep Foundation's 2005 Poll, March 29, 2005, http://www.talkaboutsleep.com/sleep–disorders/2005/04/insomnia–nsf–poll.htm (accessed February 17, 2010).

7. ResMed, Healthy Sleep, "What is Sleep Apnea?" http://www.healthysleep.com/trouble–sleeping/what–is–sleep–apnea.php (accessed February 16, 2012).

8. WebMd, "Sleep Apnea," March 2, 2010, http://www.webmd.com/sleep-disorders/sleep-apnea/sleep-apnea (accessed February 16, 2012).

9. American Sleep Apnea Association, "Do I Have Sleep Apnea?" slee-papnea.org/do-i-have-sleep-apnea.html (accessed February 16, 2012).

10. Roy H. Lubit, "Sleep Disorders," Medscape, www.emedicine.medscape.com/article/287104-overview (accessed February 10, 2012).

11. D. F. Dinges, F. Pack, K. Williams et al., "Cumulative Sleepiness, Mood Disturbance, and Psychomotor Vigilance Performance Decrements During a Week of Sleep Restricted to 4–5 Hours Per Night," *Sleep* 20, no. 4 (1997): 267–77.

12. M. Sivak, "Sleeping More as a Way to Lose Weight," *Obesity Reviews* 7, no. 3 (2006): 295–6.

13. K. Spiegel, R. Leproult, M. L'hermite-Balériaux et al., "Leptin Levels Are Dependent on Sleep Duration: Relationships with Sympathovagal Balance, Carbohydrate Regulation, Cortisol, and Thyrotropin," *The Journal of Clinical Endocrinology & Metabolism* 89, no. 11 (2004): 5762–71.

14. C. Benedict, S. J. Brooks, O. G. O'Daly et al., "Acute Sleep Deprivation Enhances the Brain's Response to Hedonic Food Stimuli: An FMRI Study," *The Journal of Clinical Endocrinology & Metabolism* 97, no. 3 (2012).

15. National Sleep Foundation, "2002 Adult Sleep Habits," March 2012, www.sleepfoundation.org/article/sleep-america-polls/2002-adult-sleep-habits, (accessed February 16, 2012). 16.   Larry Scherwitz and Deborah Kesten, "Seven Eating Styles Linked to Overeating, Overweight, and Obesity," *Explore: The Journal of Science and Healing* 1, no. 5 (2005): 342–59.

17. P. J. Shaw, "Thermoregulatory Changes, Sleep Deprivation," *Basice Science, Physiology, and Behavior*, ed. C. Kushida (New York: Marcel Kekker 2005).

18. J. J. Reilly, J. Armstrong, A. R. Dorosty et al., "Early Life Risk Factors for Obesity in Childhood: Cohort Study," *British Medical Journal* 330, no. 7504 (2005): 1357–64.

19. W. S. Agras, L. D. Hammer, F. McNicholas et al., "Risk Factors for Childhood Overweight: A Prospective Study from Birth to 9.5 Years," *The Journal of Pediatrics* 145, no. 1 (2004): 20–5.

20. Rensselaer Polytechnic Institute, Red Orbit, "Exposure To Early Evening Sunlight In Spring Creates Teenage Night Owls," July 27, 2010, http://www.redorbit.com/news/health/1896316/exposure_to_early_evening_sunlight_in_spring_creates_teenage_night/ (accessed February 16, 2012).

21. West Virginia University School of Medicine, "WVU Study Shows Too Much, Too Little Sleep Can Lead to Heart Disease," *WVU Today*, August 5, 2010, http://wvutoday.wvu.edu/n/2010/8/5/wvu–study–shows–too–much–too–little–sleep–can–lead–to–heart–disease (accessed February 16, 2011).

22. American Academy of Sleep Medicine, "Sleep Evaluation," http://www.sleepeducation.com/SleepEval.aspx (accessed February 16, 2012).

23. Healthy Living, "Dr. Oz's BIG Sleep Tips," *Huffington Post,* February 13, 2012, www.huffingtonpost.com/dr–mehmet–oz/dr–ozs–big–sleep–tips–vid_b_422243.html (accessed Feb. 13, 2012).

24. D. F. Dinges,"Sleep Debt and Scientific Evidence," *Sleep* 27, no. 6 (2004): 1050–2.

25. Institute of Medicine, *Sleep Disorders and Sleep Deprivation: An Unmet Public Health Problem* (Washington, DC: The National Academies Press; 2006).

Chapter 11: Get Moving

1. Bruce Heller, conversation with Deborah Kesten, January 30, 2007.

2. Bruce Milliman, conversation with Deborah Kesten, January 26, 2007. S. Heller, January 30, 2007.

4. Ibid.

5. Ibid.

6. Ibid.

7. W. C. Miller, D. M. Koceja, and E. J. Hamilton, "A Meta–Analysis of the Past 25 Years of Weight Loss Research Using Diet, Exercise, or Diet Plus Exercise Intervention," *International Journal of Obesity* 21, no. 10 (1997): 941–47.

8. Peg Jordan, *The Fitness Instinct: The Revolutionary New Approach to Healthy Exercise That Is Fun, Natural, and No Sweat* (Emmaus, PA: Rodale Books, 2000); WebMD Live Events Transcript Archive, "Exercise: Get Going and Keep Going—Peg Jordan, PhD, RN," January 21, 2003, www.webmd.com/content/article/60/66933.htm (accessed February 2, 2007).

9. United States Department of Agriculture, "Inside the Pyramid: What Is Physical Activity?" MyPyramid.gov, www.mypyramid.gov/pyramid/physical_activi-tyhtml (accessed February 2, 2007).

Chapter 12: Winning Weight-Loss Strategies

1. Mireille Guiliano, author presentation at Book Passage, Corde Madera, CA, November 11, 2006; Mireille Guiliano, *French Women Don't Get Fat: The Secret of Eating for Pleasure* (New York: Knopf, 2005); Christine Aaron in conversation with author Mireille Guiliano and Oprah Winfrey, "Anti–Aging Breakthroughs," *The Oprah Winfrey Show*, May 17, 2005.

2. Ibid.

Acknowledgments

We are deeply grateful to friends and colleagues who have contributed to the rich repository of food and weight wisdom that forms *Make Weight Loss Last*. Thank you all for sharing your reflections, knowledge, and insights:

To the team at *Explore: The Journal of Science and Healing*, an interdisciplinary journal that explores the healing arts, consciousness, spirituality, environmental issues, and basic science, as all these fields relate to health, for publishing our research on the seven eating styles and their link to overeating, overweight, and obesity.

To Larry Dossey, brilliant visionary, friend, colleague, and executive editor of *Explore*, for shining his intellectual and spiritual light on our work.

To Barbara Dossey, whose pioneering work in holistic health, and extensive and scholarly research in her exceptional book Florence Nightingale: Mystic, Visionary, Healer, has been an ongoing inspiration.

To Phyllis Erling, highly skilled, thorough, and thoughtful copy-editor, for making the manuscript shine; it's been a pleasure to work with you.

To Linda Roghaar, our literary agent: we're so glad you're a kindred spirit and book aficionado.

Graphic designer Rebecca Neimark of Twenty-Six Letters... your professionalism and exceptional design skills are a true gift.

To friend and colleague Barbara Birsinger, for sharing her personal and professional knowledge about emotional eating.

To Keri Brenner, award-winning journalist and friend, for telling us about her experience with "sensory eating," and for her professional interest in our work as a path that leads to weight loss.

To Vinita Azarow, friend and "fellowette" food aficionado . . . aaahhhhh . . . your story about your after—school meals with Nonna, your Italian grandmother, warms the heart . . . always.

To Bruce Heller, dear friend and physician, who shares our interest in Integrative Medicine: we're so glad that you "grock" the concept of Enlightened Exercise and that you told us about your passion for, and personal experience with, movement and motion.

To Gerdi Weider, a brilliant and exceptional research scientist and friend, who told us about her reversing—heart—disease lifestyle research at the Preventive Medicine Research Institute in Sausalito, California, and lifestyle's link to weight.

To Bruce Milliman, friend and naturopathic physician: we appre—ciate your brilliance and contribution about naturopathy's perspec—tive on exercise.

To Cassandra Vieten, brilliant psychologist, researcher, and writer: thank you for giving us insights into "negative affect."

To Meg Jordan, a like—minded medical anthropologist and health journalist, for her unique and personalized approach to movement, motion, and exercise.

To research scientist, naturopath, and friend Leanna Standish: thank you for your helpful suggestions about "molecules of emotion" and "healing environments."

To all those we have mentioned, please know that we are honored to have had the opportunity to talk with you and to learn from you. You so eloquently shared your wisdom, insights, and expertise about the multidimensional ways in which food heals. Because of you, we have learned much about the gift that is food. And because of you, the stream of nutritional and weight wisdom continues to flow.

And to all those who contribute to the human longing to find meaning in meals.

Index

D

Dairy products 116, 117

Dansinger, Michael 55

Davidson, Richard 72

Daylight Saving Time 186, 189

Depression 74, 76, 82

Desk, eating at 98

DhuraDiClemente, Carlo 55

Dieting, traditional

  breaking the diet and 41

  failure of 50

  obsessing about food 46, 47, 49

  study of 73

  successful dieting versus 47, 49

  unrealistic goals of 50, 51, 52

  weight gain of 59

Digestion 142, 143

Dine by design 149

Dopamine 103

E

Eating disorders

  binge eating 48, 70

  disconnection from the body and, 160

  evolution of 154

  mindfulness meditation for 72

  nonspecific 48–49

Eating style questionnaire

  evaluating 43

  profiles 35

  scoring 42

  using 34–35

Eating styles. *See also* specific eating

  antidotes for xxiv, 139

overeating linked with vii, 29, 32, 34, 109

overview 147

Eggs 121

Emotional eating

  antidote for 210

  decoding program for 94

  described 31

  evolution of 91

  fine–tune feelings with food 102

  negative emotions managed with 31

  obstacles of 213

  overcoming 82, 83, 105

  personal profile 34

  strategies for transforming 213

Emotions. *See also* Negative emotions

  affect on food choices 88, 102

  being with 213

  detached awareness 74

  exercise uplifting 199–200

  fine–tuning with food 105

  food's affect on xx

  releasing 144

  suppressed 87

Endocrine disruptors

  Bisphenol A (BPA) 170

  chemical "outlaws" 168

  herbicides, exposure to 169, 172

  pesticides, exposure to 169, 172

  phthalates 168, 169, 178

Endorphins 89, 199, 200

Energy, enhancing 103

Enjoy food with others 136

The Enlightened Diet. *See also* Eating Styles

  described xxii

  e–course xxi

Eucharist 158, 163

About the Authors

Deborah Kesten, MPH, is an international nutrition researcher and educator, with a specialty in preventing and reversing obesity and heart disease. She was the nutritionist on two clinical trials for reversing heart disease lifestyle changes, and co-principal investigator on innovative research about eating styles that lead to overeating, overweight, and obesity, the results of which were published in *Explore: The Journal of Science and Healing*. With more than three hundred published nutrition and health articles, she is also the award-winning author of *Feeding the Body, Nourishing the Soul*. More recent publications include *The Healing Secrets of Food*, based on her original research; and a comprehensive e-course and program about the power of food to heal multidimensionally. Among Kesten's accomplishments are contributions to scientific books and medical journals, including the *Journal of the American Medical Association*. She is married to Larry Scherwitz, PhD. Visit Deborah at www.MakeWeightLossLast.com.

Larry Scherwitz, PhD, is an international research scientist who has specialized in mind-body research and lifestyle medicine and their link to preventing and reversing heart disease and obesity. His extensive experience initiating and directing comprehensive, sustainable, lifestyle-change programs with heart patients and their families includes directing seven lifestyle programs (four in the United States, three in Europe). Dr. Scherwitz's research—including his groundbreaking discovery linking self-involvement to risk of heart attack and death from heart attack—has been published in a plethora of prestigious medical journals, including the *Journal of the American Medical Association*, *The Lancet*, and *Psychosomatic Medicine*. He has also been director of research and co—principal investigator with Dean Ornish, MD, on his heart disease reversal research. His more recent original research reveals seven newly discovered eating styles linked to overeating, overweight, and obesity. He is married to Deborah Kesten, MPH. Visit Larry at www.MakeWeightLossLast.com.

www.ingramcontent.com/pod-product-compliance
Lightning Source LLC
Chambersburg PA
CBHW022352280326
41935CB00007B/166